Praise for *Get Inside Your Doctor's Head,* by Phillip K. Peterson, M.D.

"Dr. Peterson opens a window into how an expert physician assesses complex medical problems—and how readers can use the author's insights to understand medical thinking and improve their health."
Philip A. Pizzo, M.D., Dean, Stanford University School of Medicine

"The more complicated the world of medicine becomes, the more important it is for the patient to understand what the doctor is saying and doing—and even thinking. Dr. Peterson's book will help the patient do just that, in an enjoyable and easy-to-read way."
Lee Gutkind, author of *An Immense New Power to Heal: The Promise of Personalized Medicine*

"A bold, courageous, and essential book that should be required reading for patients and physicians alike."
Thomas Goetz, M.P.H., author of *The Decision Tree: Taking Control of Your Health in the New Era of Personalized Medicine*

"No medical jargon, just clear, down-to-earth advice. This book of Dr. Peterson's clear-headed rules should be on the shelf of every caregiver who has to decide what to do when a loved one becomes ill."
Biloine W. Young, author of *The Dutiful Son, Louis W. Hill: Life in the Shadow of the Empire Builder*

"Dr. Peterson has woven wisdom, empowerment, and practical advice into a 'can't put it down' book that guides us as we make medical decisions for ourselves and our loved ones."
Michael T. Osterholm, Ph.D., M.P.H., Director, Center for Infectious Disease Research and Policy, Professor of Public Health, University of Minnesota

A Johns Hopkins Press Health Book

Get Inside Your Doctor's Head

10 Commonsense Rules for Making Better Decisions about Medical Care

Phillip K. Peterson, M.D.

The Johns Hopkins University Press • *Baltimore*

Note to the reader. This is a book of general guidance to help you work together with your physician to make your own best medical decisions. It is not intended to be used to diagnose or treat any symptom, illness, or condition. If you have a symptom, illness, or condition, please consult a qualified health care professional.

© 2013 Phillip K. Peterson
All rights reserved. Published 2013
Printed in the United States of America on acid-free paper
9 8 7 6 5 4 3 2 1

The Johns Hopkins University Press
2715 North Charles Street
Baltimore, Maryland 21218-4363
www.press.jhu.edu

Library of Congress Cataloging-in-Publication Data

Peterson, Phillip K.
     Get inside your doctor's head : ten commonsense rules for making better
decisions about medical care / Phillip K. Peterson, M.D.
          pages   cm — (A Johns Hopkins Press health book ; 33)
     ISBN-13: 978-1-4214-1069-2 (hardcover : alk. paper)
     ISBN-10: 1-4214-1069-9 (hardcover : alk. paper)
     ISBN-13: 978-1-4214-1070-8 (electronic)
     ISBN-10: 1-4214-1070-2 (electronic)
     1. Patient education. 2. Patient participation. 3. Medicine—Decision making.
4. Physician and patient. I. Title.
     R727.4.P46 2013
     613—dc23   2012050895

A catalog record for this book is available from the British Library.

*Special discounts are available for bulk purchases of this book. For more information,
please contact Special Sales at 410-516-6936 or specialsales@press.jhu.edu.*

The Johns Hopkins University Press uses environmentally friendly book materials,
including recycled text paper that is composed of at least 30 percent post-consumer
waste, whenever possible.

To Karin, Kirstin, and Per

Believe nothing, no matter where you read it or who has said it, not even if I have said it, unless it agrees with your own reason and your own common sense.

—Buddha (563–483 BCE)

Contents

Get Inside Your Doctor's Head

Applying and Breaking the Rules

I am an infectious disease doctor. I treat people who are sick with diseases that spread from one person to another person or, in some cases—such as swine flu—from an animal to a person. In the forty years since I took the Hippocratic Oath, the medical world has been transformed through breathtaking advances in medical science. And the wider world has seen a transformation, too: computer and Internet technology have put a wealth of information at everyone's fingertips. While access to this information can be extremely helpful, many of my patients find it daunting, if not overwhelming. They need tools to simplify their medical decisions. This book provides such tools, called the Ten Rules of Internal Medicine.

The Rules provide simple direction whenever a patient or family member is faced with a medical decision. Originally intended to help simplify doctors' decisions, they are equally helpful for laypeople. You can turn to them when you are weighing your doctor's recommendations about diagnostic tests and treatments. They can also help you communicate more effectively with your doctor.

When I completed internal medicine training in 1975, decision making was simple. By and large, patients trusted their doctors to make the right decisions for them. During my training, I was told by a respected internist that most of the patients who came to his office were "the worried well." By this he meant they had nothing seriously wrong with them.

Today, these two things haven't changed. Most people still trust in their doctors and are worried when they see their doctors, whether they feel well or ill. What has changed is the process of decision making—and it has changed dramatically. The authoritarian approach of "your doctor knows best" is gone. Fortunately, we are in an era of shared decision making.

Yet, paradoxically, as science advances, so does the difficulty of making medical decisions: we know more, and there are more options to consider. Furthermore, because information is instantaneously available via the Internet, patients are awash in information, both reliable and not reliable. For these reasons, making decisions about health care has become a nightmare for many people.

To help patients, some hospitals now provide decision-making services, including decision-making coaches. By revealing the complexity of medical decisions, however, these efforts sometimes make matters worse. When we have too much information, our ability to make the best decision may actually deteriorate.

This book will help simplify your medical decisions. It is built upon two premises. First, knowing something about how your doctor arrives at recommendations is extremely

---

The Ten Rules of Internal Medicine

Rule 1. If you don't know what you're doing, don't do anything.

Rule 2. If what you're doing seems to be working, think about continuing it.

Rule 3. If what you're doing doesn't seem to be working, think about doing something else.

Rule 4. Don't agree to an invasive procedure without understanding why it's needed—and without getting a second opinion.

Rule 5. If you don't have symptoms, a doctor can't make you feel better.

Rule 6. Never trust anyone completely, especially purveyors of conventional wisdom.

Rule 7. Most things are what they seem to be, except when they're not.

Rule 8. What your doctor doesn't know could kill you.

Rule 9. Timing is everything, and sometimes time is the cure.

Rule 10. Caring is always important medicine.

---

helpful (which is why this book is called *Get Inside Your Doctor's Head*). Second, common sense, the basis for each of the Ten Rules of Internal Medicine, should guide all medical decisions.

Over the past several decades, with input from mentors in infectious diseases and from students and patients, I developed the Ten Rules.

> You cannot put the same shoe on every foot.
> Publilius Syrus (85–43 BCE)

The wording of most of the Rules is exactly the same for doctors and patients, but some (Rules 4, 5, and 8) focus on you, the patient, as the decision maker.

Your doctor knows that patients rarely fit the exact textbook description of any medical problem. Yet most guides to medical decision making are rooted in the view that decisions should be backed by solid evidence. So-called evidence-based medicine, or EBM, is grounded in the statistical analysis of data from studies of groups of patients with a given disease. But in clinical practice, we rarely see a patient who perfectly fits the description of a group of patients. As Jerome Groopman observes in his book *How Doctors Think*, "Statistics cannot substitute for the human being before you." Thus, your doctor's assessment and recommendations should be based not only on EBM but also on your clinical, emotional, cultural, and social circumstances.

As with all rules, the Ten Rules of Internal Medicine have occasional exceptions—and when evidence suggests that you are such an exception, the relevant Rule should be broken. In each chapter of this book, I describe circumstances that fit the relevant Rules, as well as more unusual circumstances that necessitate breaking them.

The Ten Rules may also be useful when you are faced with nonmedical decisions. I provide some illustrations of how the Rules can help in everyday life.

About the Cases in This Book

Each chapter begins with a story of a patient from my medical practice that speaks to the corresponding Rule. (To protect confidentiality, patients' names and some of the clinical details have been changed. The one exception is where I was the patient.)

In each case, you will see how important a patient's signs and symptoms are in shaping the thinking of doctors.

Signs and symptoms are the keys to making a diagnosis—that is, figuring out what is wrong. Also, signs and symptoms forecast what will probably happen with an illness—what doctors call its prognosis.

Signs are what a physician detects when examining a patient—for example, high body temperature (fever), tenderness to touch, swelling, redness, or a rash. Some of these signs—blood pressure, pulse, rate of breathing, and temperature—are called *vital signs*. They are measured at the beginning of any physical exam, because they are vitally important. Your vital signs also weigh heavily in your doctor's thinking about what to do or recommend.

Symptoms are what usually prompt you to see your doctor. Symptoms are associated with feeling ill—for example, fever, chills, pain, fatigue, cough, sore throat, loss of appetite, headache, and diarrhea.

Doctors are especially interested in treatment that relieves symptoms and makes you feel better. But treatment can also be aimed at reversing the signs of a disease (such as high blood pressure as a sign of hardening of the arteries), even if you have few or none of the usual symptoms.

To learn more about the infections that the patients described in this book experienced, you may want to read the disease summaries in the appendix. Although I have used infectious diseases as examples, the Ten Rules apply *to all types of medical conditions*. My main hope is that you will find these commonsense Rules as useful in making decisions as I do.

If You Don't Know What You're Doing, Don't Do Anything

Gladys Worthington, a 76-year-old retired school-teacher, woke up one morning with the worst headache of her life. When it persisted into the evening, her daughters took her to the local hospital. Although she had been the picture of health for her entire life, she now had a temperature of 101.8 degrees and was markedly confused: she couldn't remember what day it was and wasn't sure where she was. The emergency room physician promptly admitted her to the hospital.

Because it was late summer and Gladys loved walking in the woods near her cabin, her primary care doctor suspected a brain infection, West Nile virus encephalitis, which causes severe inflammation. West Nile virus is carried by mosquitoes, and Gladys's daughters were sure she had been bitten many times over the summer. West Nile virus encephalitis can be fatal, especially in elderly people; unfortunately, there is no antiviral medication to treat this type of infection.

Viral encephalitis is a serious infection. It is so serious that as soon as it is suspected, many patients are treated with the drug acyclovir. However, this antiviral drug is effective only against herpes simplex virus encephalitis, a brain infection that is usually fatal without prompt treatment.

His diagnosis of encephalitis was based on Gladys's symptoms (severe headache and confusion) and physical signs (high temperature and lack of mental clarity). West Nile virus was the suspected culprit. The doctor promptly performed a lumbar puncture to obtain a sample of cerebrospinal fluid (CSF). Examination of this fluid supported his thinking that she had some kind of encephalitis. Gladys's doctor did not think she had herpes encephalitis, but to play it safe, he started treatment with acyclovir. However, test results were negative for herpes simplex virus and, more surprisingly, for West Nile virus. Results were also negative for tick-borne infections that can cause encephalitis, such as Lyme disease.

When her condition deteriorated, Gladys was transferred to our medical center in Minneapolis. When she was admitted, her temperature was 102.6. She was deeply asleep and could barely be awakened. When she did wake up, she was markedly disoriented: she didn't remember her name and didn't even recognize her daughters. The CSF and blood tests done at her referring hospital were repeated, and again the findings were negative. Additional tests for other microbes that cause encephalitis (viruses, bacteria, and fungi) were performed, and these results were negative as well. A brain scan showed abnormalities consistent with encephalitis, but it didn't reveal the cause.

Everyone now knew that Gladys had a brain inflammation that threatened her life, but its cause was unknown. This was disconcerting for her primary care doctor and frightening for her daughters and four grandchildren, all of whom were now assembled at her bedside.

At this point Gladys's primary care doctor asked me to see her. Her temperature had climbed to 104.2, and she was now in a coma. According to her daughters, she hadn't traveled outside Minnesota; she didn't have any pets or exposure to animals; and nobody around her was sick.

Despite the negative test results, I still suspected viral encephalitis. Yet two negative results for herpes simplex virus and her brain scan findings meant this virus was unlikely to be the cause of her encephalitis. Meanwhile, she was developing evidence of kidney failure (a rare but well-known complication of acyclovir). So I recommended stopping the drug. I also recommended following Rule 1: If you don't know what you are doing, don't do anything.

On the same day I saw Gladys, a neurologist was called in. All of the negative findings for an infectious disease suggested to him that her brain inflammation was due to an autoimmune disease. This meant that her immune system was attacking her own brain cells. He recommended a high dose of a steroid to combat swelling from this kind of brain inflammation. Unfortunately, this steroid has a high likelihood of serious side effects, including interference with the immune system's ability to fight infection.

Gladys's daughters, who had watched their mother lapse into a deep coma, were understandably distraught when her primary care doctor told them that the two consultants disagreed on both the diagnosis and the treatment.

In a final attempt to determine the cause of Gladys's encephalitis, the medical team suggested a brain biopsy, and her daughters reluctantly agreed. We all hoped this neurosurgical procedure would yield the cause of her encephalitis. No such luck; the brain biopsy, too, provided no useful information.

For Gladys's daughters, life stood still. Meanwhile, behind the scenes, her primary care doctor and the consultants were also losing sleep. Should her doctor do nothing, as I recommended, because of my concern about the side effects of the steroid? Or should he treat her with the steroid to reduce inflammation from what might be a fatal autoimmune brain disease, as recommended by the neurologist?

Gladys's primary care doctor ultimately agreed with me that if this was indeed an infectious disease of the brain, a steroid could make matters worse. He chose to do nothing.

It was extremely difficult for Gladys's family to hear that, despite all the medical advances over the past fifty years, her doctor was not going to do anything. But they trusted him and accepted his decision, although they were also upset that the consulting neurologist's advice wasn't taken.

During the next four weeks in the hospital, Gladys gradually regained consciousness. With supportive care and physical therapy, her health steadily improved, and she was finally discharged and sent home. Over the next six months, she regained her normal state of good health. And, according to her daughters, the following summer she made liberal use of mosquito spray.

> To do nothing is sometimes a good remedy.
>
> Hippocrates (460–377 BCE)

If you don't know what you're doing, don't do anything is the first Rule of Internal Medicine for a reason. Because virtually all treatments carry risks, doctors need to know what they are doing before they prescribe one.

The physicians initially involved in Gladys's care all agreed that her clinical picture was highly compatible with a diagnosis of viral encephalitis. But the cause of her encephalitis never became clear. (For a discussion of encephalitis and how often its cause is *not* found, see the appendix.) Because of this, and because her condition steadily deteriorated, decision making about treatment became extremely unsettling for her doctors as well as for her family.

> There are some remedies worse than the disease.
>
> Publilius Syrus (85–43 BCE)

The origin of Rule 1 lies with Hippocrates, the father of Western medicine, whose oath is still taken by medical students at graduation: "I swear . . . I will use regimens for the benefit of the ill in accordance with my ability and my judgment, but from [what is] to their harm or injustice I will keep [them]." The primary responsibility of a doctor is not to make matters worse. The well-known phrase "first, do no harm" (*Primum non nocere*) is credited to the seventeenth-century physician Thomas Sydenham.

RULE
1

That virtually all forms of treatment carry risks is at the heart of Rule 1. It also explains why evidence-based research (designed to identify the risks as well as benefits of treatments) is crucial for good medical decisions.

Historically, Western medicine has been guided by the view that any therapeutic recommendation should be based on evidence that it actually works. Our concept of what constitutes "evidence-based medicine" underwent a marked transformation in the 1990s (more on this topic in the discussion of Rule 2). In Gladys's case, there was no evidence to support the use of a steroid. However, plenty of evidence exists that steroids can be harmful.

Applying Rule 1

Don't just do something, stand there.
Peter Ustinov (1921–2004)

Gladys's primary care doctor followed Rule 1. He was aware that we didn't know what we were dealing with, so he didn't want to subject her to the risks of a steroid.

Should you find yourself in the uncomfortable shoes of Gladys's daughters—or, if you yourself are sick—don't just swallow hard and stay silent.

- If your doctor advises doing nothing, ask why.
- Ask about the evidence for and against withholding treatment.

- Ask about all the other potential options. For each option, ask about the potential benefits and risks.

A good doctor will welcome these questions. In fact, in our era of shared decision making, your doctor expects you to speak up. And, as they were in Gladys's case, family members sometimes are in the best position to ask questions.

In my role as an infectious diseases consultant, I often have to admit I don't understand the cause of a patient's problem. Paradoxically, confessing my ignorance has become more common as my experience with patients like Gladys has grown. Often the most useful function I play as a consultant is to allay a primary care doctor's fear that he or she has overlooked an important test or treatment.

In difficult cases, medical decisions are commonly made with great humility. I have found that confessing my ignorance is often appreciated—not only by physicians, but also by patients and their families, so long as I explain my thinking.

Over the years, I also have learned to apply Rule 1 in making many nonmedical decisions as well. For example, I never try to fix a running toilet or a leaking roof, as I have learned from experience that I can indeed make these matters worse. And with many a difficult but nonpressing practical decision, I have found that sleeping on it resolves the problem. As with Gladys's encephalitis, nature often takes care of the matter.

Breaking Rule 1

When is it necessary to do something in the face of ignorance and uncertainty? *When doing nothing is likely to result in death or serious harm.*

Encephalitis caused by herpes simplex virus often causes severe brain damage. But unlike almost all other viral infections of the nervous system, herpes encephalitis can be treated. Thus, the antiviral drug acyclovir should be started in all cases when herpes simplex is considered a possible cause of encephalitis. The reason for such early therapy is based on clear evidence that a delay in treatment increases the likelihood of death if the cause is indeed herpes simplex. And, as in Gladys's case, acyclovir can be stopped if the test findings for the virus prove negative.

Most medical decisions are based on estimates of the consequences of our actions (or inactions). Before you decide to break Rule 1 by doing something in the face of uncertainty, *make sure you and your doctor have discussed and weighed the evidence together.* Good, clear communication is crucial. As physicians Leora Horwitz and Allan Detsky note, "In the end, patients need to be absolutely confident that their physician knows everything of importance about them, no matter who that physician is."

If What You're Doing Seems to Be Working, Think about Continuing It

Like many Minnesotans, Ted Schmidt, a 48-year-old farmer from Pipestone, spent his winters in Arizona. Unlike most Minnesotans, however, he traveled with someone else's kidney. Because of chronic kidney failure caused by glomerulonephritis, he had received a kidney transplant at the University of Minnesota Medical Center three years earlier. Except for a brief bout of transplant rejection, he had done remarkably well. To prevent rejection of his transplanted kidney, he was taking medications that suppressed his immune system. He also took an antibiotic called sulfisoxazole. The week before he left for Arizona in December, he decided on his own to stop taking the sulfisoxazole.

During his first several weeks in Arizona, Ted felt perfectly fine. He and his wife went hiking almost daily in the nearby desert. In February, however, Ted developed a cough he couldn't shake. He also had a fever, lost his appetite, and felt exhausted. When he began coughing up blood, his wife decided it was time for him to return to Minnesota for a medical evaluation.

Ted's history of coughing up blood, coupled with the fact that he was taking potent immunosuppressive drugs, prompted his immediate admission to the University of Minnesota Medical Center Kidney Transplant Service. On admission, Ted's temperature was 102.5 degrees, and his breathing and pulse were rapid. When the admitting doctor examined his lungs with a stethoscope, she heard a crackly sound over the right side of his chest. Her gentle thumping of this area indicated the presence of fluid. Ted's doctor ordered a chest x-ray, which showed that Ted had fluid between his right lung and chest wall. Also, there was an abscess in his right lung. It was now clear that the cause of Ted's cough and fever lay in his right lung. His doctor took a sample of the fluid and sent it to the lab to test for microbes that cause lung infections in people who have had a kidney transplant.

This is when I was called in. I knew Ted was at greatest risk for an infection caused by microbes called "opportunists." Opportunists are so named because they take advantage of people who have a weakened immune system. In Ted's case, the medications he was taking to prevent the rejection of his transplanted kidney had impaired his immune system's defenses against these microbes. Ted's travel to Arizona placed him at risk for a particular opportunistic fungus. When the winds blow in certain deserts of the Southwest, spores of this fungus circulate. Anyone can inhale them without realizing it, but if they land in the lung of someone whose defenses are weakened, the person can come down with a life-threatening fungal infection.

Ted's travel to Arizona, his symptoms of fever and coughing up blood, and his signs of lung infection on the physical exam and chest x-ray all fit the diagnosis of this opportunistic fungal infection. The medical resident on our infectious diseases consultation team disagreed with me. He thought this was some kind of bacterial infection.

When the test results came in, to my chagrin the resident turned out to be right. Ted's travel to Arizona was a "red herring": it had nothing to do with his illness, which turned out to be nocardiosis, an opportunistic bacterial (rather than fungal) infection.

One of the reasons I didn't think of nocardiosis was that, until then, I hadn't seen a single case in a kidney transplant patient. When I discussed Ted's case with Richard Simmons, a world-renowned transplant surgeon, he wasn't surprised. In 1973, he explained, transplant doctors at the University of Minnesota started the routine use of sulfisoxazole—the antibiotic Ted decided to stop taking—for transplant recipients. As a result, this bacterial infection essentially disappeared. Because Ted was no longer taking the drug, he became vulnerable to this infection. Sulfisoxazole worked beautifully, and there was very good reason for Ted to keep taking it. He didn't, and he paid the price of not following Rule 2: If what you're doing seems to be working, think about continuing it.

I prescribed a high dose of sulfisoxazole, and after Ted had spent a week in the hospital, his cough and fever subsided. I assured him and his wife that he was likely to recover completely but slowly. This time he didn't miss any doses of his sulfisoxazole, and by the next winter he was back to good health.

Practice is the best of all instructors.

Publilius Syrus (85–43 BCE)

In the 1990s, randomized clinical trials (RCTs) became the gold standard of evidence-based medicine (EBM). From that time on, all medical trainees and practitioners have been urged to "think EBM." Thus, to understand your doctor's thinking, it is useful for you to know something about RCTs.

Randomized clinical trials are studies aimed at determining the safety and efficacy of new treatments. Patients who volunteer for these studies are randomly assigned to separate groups that will be used to compare different treatments. Neither the researchers nor the patients are allowed to choose the group a patient is assigned to. In this way, clinical factors that often influence the response to a treatment—age, gender, severity of illness, and so on—are balanced among the treatment groups.

In some RCTs, an active drug is compared with a placebo. A placebo is an inactive substance—often called a sugar pill—disguised to look just like the active drug. In what are called double-blind, placebo-controlled RCTs, neither the researchers nor the patients know what each patient receives—either the real drug or the placebo—until the study is completed.

Yet there is much more to health care than EBM and controlled clinical trials. Doctors also heavily rely on their own clinical experience ("experience-based medicine"). Generally speaking, this is especially true for surgeons. If, in their experience, a surgical procedure (or a medication) works, they will think twice before recommending something else. In short, doctors are reluctant to change what they are doing if their patients are doing well. (For more about infections in transplant patients and the benefit of antibiotics such as sulfisoxazole, see the appendix.)

Applying Rule 2

If it ain't broke, don't fix it.

Bert Lance (1931–)

Rule 2 applies to all forms of medication—drugs that help with your blood pressure, cholesterol, diabetes, arthritis, heart failure, and so on. If what your doctor prescribes appears to be working, continue with the recommended course of treatment. This recommendation can be especially important for antibiotics. For example, if you're supposed to take an antibiotic for four weeks and you feel well after two, continue the antibiotic for the full four weeks. Stopping the antibiotic before you have taken the full course can lead to antibiotic-resistant infections.

Failing to take medications as prescribed is an enormous and very expensive problem. According to a World Health Organization fact sheet, most patients fail to take their medications correctly. And according to the *New York Times*, such lapses result in more than $100 billion in costs for unnecessary hospitalizations each year.

I never learned why Ted Schmidt stopped taking sulfisoxazole. Possibly, the benefits and risks weren't adequately explained to him in terms he could easily understand. Don't let this happen to you.

- Ask your doctor why he or she recommends continuing any particular medication or treatment.
- Make sure you understand exactly how long the treatment or course of medication will be.
- Ask what other options are available.
- Ask about the potential benefits, risks, and side effects of each option.
- Before you stop taking any medication earlier than prescribed, speak with your doctor, and make sure you understand the potential consequences.

Breaking Rule 2

Rule 2 should be broken when the evidence suggests that the side effects and risks of continuing a treatment or course of medication begin to outweigh the benefits.

A good example is the antibiotic trovafloxacin. Approved in 1998 by the U.S. Food and Drug Administration (FDA), trovafloxacin was shown to be highly effective in treating pneumonia and many other infections. In early studies of more than five thousand patients, no serious toxicity appeared.

Because of trovafloxacin's excellent track record in treating a wide variety of infections, within less than a year after its approval, more than one million patients had been treated with it. Soon, however, a serious, unanticipated problem emerged. The drug proved toxic to some people's livers. Although this side effect was rare, occurring in fewer than one in ten thousand patients, the FDA widely restricted the drug's use. Today it is no longer used at all.

Doctors need to know that a treatment isn't worse than the illness. Similarly, you need to know that the potential side effects of a drug don't outweigh the benefits, even if you are doing well on the medication. If, after a thorough discussion with your doctor, you aren't convinced of this, consider breaking Rule 2.

. . . because that's where the money is.

Willie Sutton (1901–1980)

Ted Schmidt's case not only serves as a good example of Rule 2 of Internal Medicine but also speaks to Sutton's Law, another valuable tool in medical decision making. Unlike the Rules, however, physicians *never* break Sutton's Law.

Sutton's Law is named after an infamous and highly successful bank robber, Willie "The Actor" Sutton. After he was apprehended, he allegedly was asked by a reporter, "Why do you rob banks?" Incredulous, he pointed out that banks are where the money is.

Sutton's Law first appeared in the medical literature in the journal *Medicine* in 1961, in a now classic article titled "Fever of Undetermined Origin." The authors, Robert Petersdorf and

Paul Beeson, proposed that Sutton's Law be applied whenever deciding what diagnosis to consider first. In medicine, of course, Sutton's Law means, "Go first where the symptoms and signs are pointing you." For doctors, this means taking a detailed history and doing a thorough physical exam.

In Ted Schmidt's case, for example, he had a cough with bloody sputum. A physical exam and a chest x-ray determined that he had fluid in his lung. Thus, his doctor promptly took a sample of the fluid and established the diagnosis.

Sutton's Law has proved invaluable not only in evaluating patients with a history of prolonged fever but also in prioritizing diagnostic possibilities for all medical conditions. Applying Sutton's Law saves time (by helping doctors zero in on the right treatment) and money (by eliminating needless tests).

If What You're Doing Doesn't Seem to Be Working, Think about Doing Something Else

One morning, 7-year-old Molly Aronson awoke with pain in her right hip. Understandably, her mother was very worried, especially when Molly developed a shaking chill and felt, to her mother's touch, as if she were burning up. She also limped because her pain was so severe.

Until then, Molly had been a healthy, vivacious child. Despite her symptoms, she wanted to go to that day's session of summer camp. But her mother knew this problem needed immediate medical attention and brought her to the emergency room at our medical center.

The ER doctor suspected a hip infection and called for an orthopedic surgery consultant. Both agreed that Molly probably had an acute septic (infected) arthritis of the right hip. After swabbing the skin over the hip with an antiseptic and administering a local anesthetic, the orthopedist withdrew some fluid through a syringe for assessment by the clinical microbiology lab.

The tests revealed clusters of bacteria and many white blood cells. These findings supported the suspicion of Molly's doctors that she had septic arthritis caused by a bacterium called *Staphylococcus aureus*. Molly was admitted to the pediatric service and immediately treated with cefazolin, a tried-and-true antibiotic for this kind of infection.

During that first day in the hospital, however, her condition worsened. Yet the next day, the results of the culture of the hip fluid, and of a blood sample, confirmed that this was indeed a *Staphylococcus aureus* infection.

I was then called in as an infectious diseases consultant to see Molly.

Molly's mom and dad were both at her bedside, and it was apparent they hadn't slept a wink. Molly was sleepy but, given the circumstances, surprisingly cheerful. She had been taken to the operating room, where her hip had been opened and the pus drained. But she was still in pain, had a temperature of 103 degrees, and looked very sick.

Even though everything that needed to be done had been done up to this point, it was time to apply Rule 3: If what you're doing doesn't seem to be working, think about doing something else. A different antibiotic was in order. I recommended changing to vancomycin.

Soon after I saw Molly, the results of another test were reported to her pediatrician. Surprisingly, the test showed that the *Staphylococcus aureus* in Molly's hip and bloodstream was resistant to cefazolin as well as to related antibiotics. Like almost all *Staphylococcus aureus* strains, however, it was sensitive to the antibiotic vancomycin. Sadly, although her therapy had already been changed to this antibiotic, her condition continued to deteriorate.

This is when my pediatric infectious diseases colleague took over as the consultant. Unfortunately, by this time, her infection had progressed, and Molly's vital organs were failing. On the third day of her hospitalization, she developed respiratory failure. She was transferred to the pediatric critical care unit and put on a respirator. After five agonizing weeks of intensive treatment for acute respiratory distress syndrome and severe pneumonia, Molly died of a pulmonary hemorrhage.

> Hindsight is always twenty-twenty.
>
> Billy Wilder (1906–2002)

When I saw Molly, I was deeply concerned by how severe her illness was. But I was astonished to learn that her infection was caused by methicillin-resistant *Staphylococcus aureus* (MRSA). Molly's case was one of the first in an epidemic that became known as community-associated MRSA (CA-MRSA). (To read more about MRSA, see the appendix.)

The problem of antibiotic resistance is not limited to *Staphylococcus aureus*. Many other bacterial species have developed strategies to circumvent antibiotics. As a rule, the emergence of such resistance is due to "antibiotic pressure," fueled by the overuse and misuse of antibiotics. This is a good example of Darwinian survival of the fittest: in the presence of an antibiotic, the bacteria that survive are fit to survive because they are resistant to the antibiotic—thus, only the fit survive, reproduce, and give rise to additional generations of resistant bacteria.

In the 1970s and 1980s, the pharmaceutical industry developed many antibiotics to combat resistance of bacteria that are classified as "gram-negative." These drugs worked well for some years. Then, in the 1990s, antibiotic-resistant "gram-positive" bacteria, such as MRSA and *Streptococcus pneumoniae* (the most important cause of pneumonia), emerged. As a result, there was a flurry of activity to develop antibiotics active against these bacteria. But by the end of the twentieth century, the pharmaceutical industry's pipeline of new antibiotics had largely dried up.

We now face a serious situation where we have no effective antibiotics for certain kinds of bacterial infections. The solution to this problem is complex, but one thing is clear: physicians and patients need to work together to limit antibiotic overuse and misuse.

> Errors in judgment must occur in the practice of an art which consists of balancing possibilities.
>
> Sir William Osler (1849–1919)

I wasn't involved in the initial decision to prescribe cefazolin for Molly. In 1997, when Molly's illness occurred, this was the right antibiotic to start with. There was no reason to suspect MRSA at the time. In hindsight, however, once the antibiotic-susceptibility test results were known, this turned out to be a fatal error. Usually we physicians have time to correct our bad calls and errors, and the patient recovers. But in

Molly's case, by the time her antibiotic was changed, it was too late.

What sets such errors of judgment apart from medical malpractice is something called the standard of care: what most doctors would do given the same set of circumstances. Once CA-MRSA became widespread, at the turn of the century, the standard of care changed. Now, in any case when a serious *Staphylococcus aureus* infection is suspected, initial antibiotic treatment should be aimed at potential MRSA.

Applying Rule 3

If you do not change direction, you may end up where you are heading.

Lao Tzu (551–479 BCE)

In any given year, most of us develop at least one infection. If an infection is serious enough that you see your doctor, and if your doctor believes that your infection is bacterial, he or she may recommend an antibiotic—a drug that acts against bacteria. (Antibiotics shouldn't be prescribed for other types of microorganisms, such as viruses—the cause of the common cold—and infectious fungi.) Your doctor is familiar with the many different kinds of bacterial infections and knows which antibiotics work (and don't work).

As in Molly's case, we doctors usually don't know at first which bacterium is causing the illness. At this early stage, therapy is called "empiric"—that is, based on the most likely

RULE
3

bacterium. When lab results come back, your doctor may then reconsider the initial antibiotic choice. However, if your condition doesn't improve, no matter what the lab tests reveal, your doctor needs to think about Rule 3.

If you (or a loved one) are being treated for any medical problem and the condition keeps getting worse, proceed as follows:

- Ask your doctor whether another treatment might work better—and find out what all the other possible options are.
- Ask for a second medical opinion—that is, see a doctor with expertise related to your specific problem. (Two heads are often better than one, especially when things get complicated.) For example, if the problem involves your lungs, see a lung specialist. If it involves you heart, consult a heart specialist.

Rule 3 can also be valuable in making many nonmedical decisions. Knowing when to change course can avoid a lot of emotional turmoil or financial woe—a lesson I have learned more than once.

Breaking Rule 3

As an internist, I care mainly for adults, and I am much more familiar with the health issues of seniors than those of children such as Molly. With the exception of HIV/AIDS, most life-threatening infections in the United States occur in people over 65. Pneumonia is the most common fatal infectious disease worldwide, and a particular problem among the elderly.

Some years ago, I was part of a team that conducted a randomized clinical trial comparing two antibiotics for patients who developed pneumonia in nursing homes. Internal medicine residents cared for the patients in this trial. Typically, if their patients still had a fever after two days of an antibiotic, many of the residents wanted to follow Rule 3 and change to a different antibiotic.

As the most experienced member of our team knew, however, elderly folks often take longer to respond to treatment. Thus, we persuaded the residents not to change antibiotics just because of persistent fever, if a patient was otherwise doing well. At the end of the study, we determined that it took an average of four days for fever to break in these elderly patients, and almost all of them recovered fully. Just as we anticipated, it made sense to break Rule 3 as long as the overall condition of the patients was taken into account.

Don't Agree to an Invasive Procedure without Understanding Why It's Needed—and without Getting a Second Opinion

When Awa Fahia, a 28-year-old immigrant from Somalia, arrived in Minneapolis, she had never seen snow and was not prepared for temperatures well below zero. However, with the help of family members already acclimated to Minnesota, she made the best of it. Anything seemed better than the war-torn country and the refugee camp she had left behind.

Awa was three months pregnant with her first child when she arrived in Minneapolis. Her pregnancy went well, and in July she delivered a healthy baby boy at our medical center.

In September, while standing in line at the grocery store, Awa had a seizure. She didn't have a history of epilepsy, so this seizure was entirely unexpected—and very frightening. An ambulance was called, and Awa was brought to our emergency room.

By the time she arrived in the ER she had recovered. Through a Somali interpreter, the ER physician learned that

Awa had been having increasingly severe headaches for the past week. Otherwise, she was healthy, and the ER doctor's exam didn't find any problems. However, a CT (computed tomography) scan of her brain revealed a large mass in the right frontal lobe.

Given her history and the brain scan findings, Awa was admitted to the Neurosurgery Service for a brain biopsy. With the help of an interpreter, the neurosurgical resident confirmed her history. His exam, however, detected weakness in her left leg. He ordered an MRI (magnetic resonance imaging) scan of her brain. It, too, showed a large mass in the frontal lobe.

Awa's neurosurgeons were almost certain she had a glioblastoma, a type of brain cancer that is usually fatal. They scheduled her for surgery to obtain a piece of brain tissue for examination by pathologists.

Because Awa was from Somalia, where certain kinds of brain infection are more common than elsewhere, I was asked to see her. With the help of a Somali interpreter, I learned that several of her family members had been treated in the refugee camp for tuberculosis (TB). But Awa believed she had been screened for TB in the camp and that the results were negative. Other than frequent headaches and the single seizure episode, she had no symptoms. Findings from routine laboratory tests, including a chest x-ray, were normal.

When I reviewed Awa's MRI scan, I was impressed by the size and the nasty appearance of the brain mass. It certainly looked like a glioblastoma. But because Awa was from Somalia, TB needed to be considered. I suggested a TB skin test; if it were negative in forty-eight hours, this would be evidence against TB. I felt strongly that this was a situation that called for Rule 4: Don't agree to an invasive procedure without understanding why it's needed—and without getting a second opinion.

I urged Awa's neurosurgeons to put off the biopsy until we knew the result of her TB skin test. Despite my recommendation, a brain biopsy was performed the next day.

When the report from the surgical pathologist came back, it revealed no cancer. But it did reveal "multiple granulomas and acid fast bacilli"—in other words, TB.

The diagnosis was now clear: Awa had TB of the central nervous system. I recommended the antibiotics that are usually used to treat this infection. Because her chest x-ray showed no abnormality, there was no reason to worry about her spreading TB to others.

Awa's postoperative recovery was uneventful. After being discharged from the hospital, she attended our TB clinic. After nine months of antibiotic treatment, she was cured.

There is no such thing as minor surgery, but there are a lot of minor surgeons.

Harvey Cushing (1869–1939)

Originally, Rule 4, addressed to doctors, was *Keep your patients out of the hands of surgeons at all costs.* By the end of the twentieth century, it was clear that Rule 4 needed to be changed: *Don't agree to an invasive procedure without understanding why it's needed—and without getting a second opinion.*

This modification became necessary because a number of subspecialists in internal medicine were routinely carrying out invasive procedures—defined as procedures that literally get under the skin or inside the body. Cardiologists routinely were doing coronary angioplasties, gastroenterologists regularly performed colonoscopies, and pulmonologists commonly did bronchoscopies. Invasive radiologists got into the act when they began puncturing the skin to biopsy tissues or drain abscesses.

The essential point of Rule 4 is that all invasive procedures carry risks. As suggested by Harvey Cushing, the founding father of modern neurosurgery, choosing the right surgeon is of paramount importance. But for the primary care doctor, the first question is, should surgery or any other invasive procedure be considered at all?

In the case of Awa, a Somali immigrant with a mass in her brain, a malignancy wasn't the first thing to think of. And surgery wasn't the first diagnostic test to consider. Central nervous system TB, the cause of her brain mass, is treated with antibiotics; surgical removal or drainage isn't needed. (For a discussion of TB, see the appendix.)

If Awa had been born in Minnesota rather than Somalia, a brain tumor would most likely have been the correct diagnosis. But in Somalia, TB is still pervasive.

In teaching medical students how to prioritize potential diagnoses, we use the adage, "When you hear hoof beats, think of horses, not zebras." In other words, "Common things are common." However, when a patient recently emigrated from

East Africa, where zebras are common, think of zebras, not horses.

For a close look at modern-day surgery, I recommend Atul Gawande's books *Complications: A Surgeon's Notes on an Imperfect Science* and *The Checklist Manifesto*. According to Dr. Gawande, the average American has seven operations in his or her lifetime. Surgeons perform more than fifty million operations in the United States each year. Although surgery goes well most of the time, there are more than five million surgical complications per year.

For many medical conditions, surgery is the clear treatment of choice. And, in some situations, surgery is lifesaving.

Applying Rule 4

Stay out of harm's way.

Rule 4 underscores the importance of paying serious attention whenever your doctor recommends surgery—or any other invasive procedure. Here are some questions you should ask:

- Is this invasive strategy really necessary? Why?
- Is this the best way to treat my condition? Why?
- Are there any noninvasive treatments? If so, how effective are they? What are the potential risks and side effects of each one?

If surgery or some other invasive procedure is in fact the best (or the only good) option, it's important to ask these questions as well:

RULE
4

- How long will it take?
- Where will it be done?
- What are the potential risks?
- How long will recovery take?
- Which surgeon would you go to if you (or your mother, father, or child) needed this operation? Why?

Not surprisingly, the doctors with the most experience in performing a particular procedure generally have the best outcomes.

Unless your problem demands immediate intervention, you will have time to carefully consider your options and the answers you get to these questions. Also, don't be afraid to get a second medical opinion.

Breaking Rule 4

Hagos Yakob, an 8-year-old boy, was admitted to our medical center one month after emigrating from Ethiopia to Minnesota. Except for a history of malaria in his home country, he had been a healthy child.

When he developed a fever, his parents thought this was another bout of malaria and brought him to our ER. While malaria was high on the ER doctor's list of diagnostic possibilities, she was most concerned by Hagos's complaint of pain in the left side of his abdomen. When she examined his abdomen, she found an enlarged and tender spleen. X-rays revealed that the spleen was markedly swollen and contained a large pocket of pus (called an abscess).

On admission to the pediatrics service, Hagos had a temperature of 104.2 degrees, his pulse and his breathing were rapid, and his blood pressure was disturbingly low (90/60). Because neither Hagos nor his parents spoke English, an Ethiopian interpreter was called in. Through the interpreter it was learned that Hagos had been sick for about a week. His main symptoms were fever, shaking chills, loss of appetite, and pain in the upper left side of his abdomen. A second physical exam confirmed an enlarged spleen that was tender to the touch. Because the clinical picture looked like septic shock, a highly fatal condition, Hagos was transferred to the pediatric intensive care unit.

An intravenous antibiotic had been started in the ER. Given the severity of Hagos's infection and his country of origin, the pediatric critical care physician added a second antibiotic to make sure all infectious bacteria would be killed off. A surgical consultant was also called in for advice about possible surgery for the abscess in Hagos's spleen.

Although an enlarged spleen commonly occurs with malaria, an abscess was unlikely. Nonetheless, a smear of Hagos's blood was taken, to check for the malaria parasite. The test results came back negative. Both the pediatrician and the surgical consultant agreed that the abscess in the spleen pointed to a bacterial infection that needed surgical attention some time soon.

By the next morning, the blood sample taken in the ER was growing a dangerous bacterium. It was identified as *Salmonella typhi*, the microbe that causes typhoid fever.

RULE
4

Although Hagos was receiving antibiotics active against this bacterium, his clinical condition remained grave. This is when I was called in to see him. By this time, he had been placed on a medicine to raise his blood pressure, and it was barely working. Both parents were at his bedside trying to comfort him. Through an interpreter, I tried my best to allay their anxiety, while at the same time letting them know this was a very serious situation.

Splenic abscesses caused by *Salmonella typhi* are rare in the United States. But I knew from reading the medical literature that they are usually fatal if the spleen isn't removed. The surgical consultant and pediatrician coordinating Hagos's care agreed.

Through the interpreter, we carefully explained to Hagos's parents the need for an immediate splenectomy. However, Hagos's father refused to permit anyone to operate on his son. In his culture, we were told, this kind of decision is made by community elders. No matter how many doctors carefully explained the need for urgent surgery, his father insisted otherwise—his father broke Rule 4.

Over the next twenty-four hours, Hagos's life hung in the balance. He continued to spike a fever, his blood pressure remained low, and he needed to be placed on a respirator. Through interpreters, several additional attempts—more like pleadings—were made to explain the extreme seriousness of the situation. With Hagos on death's doorstep, his father finally consented to surgery.

The splenectomy saved Hagos's life. Antibiotic therapy

was continued for two weeks afterward, and Hagos was cured of typhoid fever.

Although infectious diseases specialists are "noninvasive" doctors, when we see an abscess we know that the scalpel is usually the best antibiotic. A good case in point was Hagos's splenic abscess. (To read more about typhoid fever, see the appendix.) Similarly, if you have the life-threatening skin infection called necrotizing fasciitis (popularly referred to as "flesh-eating bacteria"), you need a good surgeon immediately. Unless all the dead tissue is promptly removed, you won't survive. In Hagos's case, despite the surgeon's explanation of the critical need for surgery—reinforced by second and third medical opinions—his father withheld permission to operate. Fortunately, the cultural barrier underlying his reluctance was surmounted in the nick of time.

When my son, Per, was 11 years old, our family took a vacation in Mexico. On his first school day after we returned, the school nurse called to say that Per was vomiting and had diarrhea. Although his mother initially suspected he was feigning illness to get out of school, she picked him up and brought him home. Then she called me, because he really was sick.

I'm an infectious diseases specialist, so to me the diagnosis seemed obvious: traveler's diarrhea. But when his symptoms got worse the next day, I took him to see a colleague, a pediatric infectious diseases specialist. He concurred with my diagnosis, but (wisely) also asked a surgeon to see Per. After spending less than a minute with my son, the surgeon concluded that he had appendicitis, even though he didn't have a fever or abdominal pain.

To my amazement, the surgeon found a perforated appendix. My reluctance to get a surgical opinion was based on my fear of the complications of surgery. This was another situation where it was important to follow rather than break Rule 4.

If You Don't Have Symptoms, a Doctor Can't Make You Feel Better

Thelma Moore, an 88-year-old grandmother, developed a high spiking fever and an angry-looking rash over her entire body. She had recently been treated at our hospital for a stroke, and her hospitalization was complicated by pneumonia. Also, she had lost control of her bladder, and a catheter was inserted. Pain when she urinated, plus a fever, prompted the treatment of a urinary tract infection. Despite these complications, by the end of her third week of hospitalization she was ready for discharge. Because she lived alone and was unsteady on her feet, she was transferred to a nursing home for rehabilitation.

Thelma's family was very close-knit. While she was in the hospital after having the stroke, she received daily visits from her daughter, her son, and one or more of her four grandchildren. At the time of her discharge, they were concerned about how weak she was. Also, she wasn't her usual cheery self, and her mind was no longer sharp as a tack. They wondered whether this was a result of her stroke, or could it be Alzheimer's disease?

Although Thelma received two courses of antibiotics while in the hospital, when she was admitted to the nursing home she was no longer taking any medications. The doctor on call ordered a urine culture. Her children thought this was unusual, because the catheter had been removed from her bladder a week before. Also, she didn't have any complaints to suggest that she might have an infection in her urinary tract. Nonetheless, the culture was reported as positive for a bacterium called *Klebsiella pneumoniae.*

Thelma's doctor prescribed (over the phone) a two-week course of an antibiotic. Meanwhile, the nurse made a note in Thelma's record that she wasn't having any trouble urinating and didn't have a fever.

Five days later, she developed an itchy red rash on her arms and legs. Over the next two days, the rash rapidly spread to the rest of her body. Also, she had difficulty eating because of pain when she tried to swallow. Her temperature was 101 degrees.

By the time Thelma was readmitted to our hospital, her temperature had climbed to 103.2. She had a red rash that was peeling in sheets on several areas of her body. Her mouth and throat were swollen, intensely red, and peeling. The whites of her eyes were also red. Her doctor diagnosed this as a serious allergic reaction called Stevens-Johnson syndrome. The suspected culprit was the antibiotic she had been given for her urinary tract infection—an infection for which she had tested positive, but which she showed no symptoms of having.

I was asked to see Thelma because her urine culture was positive not merely for *Klebsiella pneumoniae* but for a specific strain that is resistant to virtually all antibiotics. When the medical student on our infectious diseases consultation team presented the case to me, we talked about the recent emergence of this bacterial strain. However, the main focus of our discussion was on Rule 5: If you don't have symptoms, a doctor can't make you feel better. Why on earth was Thelma given an antibiotic when she didn't have any symptoms?

Fortunately, Thelma's doctors were able to treat the Stevens-Johnson syndrome with a steroid—thus saving her life. After Thelma's rocky two-week hospitalization, her daughter asked that she be sent home with her rather than back to the nursing home. Not every family is able to care for their loved ones at home, but Thelma's family pulled it off. It occurred to me, and probably to her children, that if she had been discharged to her daughter's home the first time, she would have been spared this frightening and costly rehospitalization.

Half of modern drugs could well be thrown out of the window, except birds might eat them.

Martin H. Fischer, M.D. (1879–1962)

An apple a day keeps the doctor away, depending upon how good your aim is.

Dale Hammerschmidt, M.D. (1946–)

Experience tempers a doctor's enthusiasm, not only for surgical interventions, but for medical treatments in general. Caution is especially important when we treat patients with no symptoms.

Symptoms of a urinary tract infection include urinating frequently, burning or pain when urinating, pain in the area over the kidney, and fever. Thelma did not have any of these symptoms. (For a discussion of this kind of urinary tract infection—called asymptomatic bacteriuria—and why it shouldn't be treated, see the appendix.) But after starting treatment with an antibiotic, Thelma did develop symptoms: a sudden, severe (fulminant) rash and fever caused by an allergic reaction to the antibiotic.

It was fortunate that Thelma's urinary tract infection was asymptomatic and not in need of treatment. The highly antibiotic-resistant bacterium causing her infection, called carbapenem-resistant *Klebsiella pneumoniae* (CRKP), has now spread in hospitals throughout the United States. As the name suggests, this bacterium is highly resistant to almost all antibiotics, including carbapenems. Until the past few years, carbapenems could be relied on to kill virtually all bacteria. Unfortunately, treatment options are extremely limited, and in some cases nonexistent, for this antibiotic-resistant microbe.

Most patients with CRKP infections—like Thelma—are elderly and have underlying medical conditions. The problem is fueled by the widespread use (and overuse) of antibiotics in hospitals. Like many hospital-associated infections, CRKP is spread from one patient to the next by the hands of hospital personnel. Solving and preventing this problem isn't difficult or high-tech. The simple maneuver of frequent hand-washing, taught to us by our mothers, can markedly reduce the risk of this and many other infections acquired in the hospital.

Applying Rule 5

> A smart mother makes often a better diagnosis than a poor doctor.
>
> August Bier (1861–1949)

As in Thelma's case, the consequences of breaking Rule 5 can be very serious. Your doctor should always have a clear, sound rationale for ordering laboratory tests or recommending medications or medical procedures. If your doctor recommends a test—especially if you have no symptoms—ask these questions:

- Why is this test necessary?
- What might happen if we don't do the test?

When you have no symptoms, and your doctor recommends a drug, procedure, or other treatment, ask these questions:

- What are the potential risks and side effects of this drug, procedure, or treatment?
- What do you believe will probably happen if I don't take this drug, or receive this treatment, or undergo this procedure?

If your doctor's reasoning doesn't make sense to you, say no to the test, medication, procedure, or treatment. Also think seriously about getting a second medical opinion.

Unfortunately, doctors can't remember all the potential side effects of every drug they prescribe. The good news is that the Internet can help. Just access www.drugs.com, where you will find a listing of all known side effects of nearly every medication.

If you are making a medical decision on behalf of a loved one, take Rule 5 especially to heart. Don't be afraid to speak up. Read Lee Gutkind's book *Silence Kills: Speaking Out and Saving Lives*, and you will never be tempted to suffer in silence again.

Communication breakdowns are at the root of most medical errors. This means most medical errors are preventable— and you can help prevent them simply by asking the right questions at the right times. Remember, good doctors want you to speak up.

And if you see hospital personnel not washing their hands before caring for someone, politely remind them to do so. Believe it or not, this reminder will probably have more of an impact if it comes from you than if it comes from a hospital coworker.

Rule 5 is also useful in many nonmedical contexts. If you currently have nothing to complain about in your personal life, be thankful. As you know, things will change.

Breaking Rule 5

Most authorities do recommend breaking Rule 5 for pregnant women with asymptomatic bacteriuria. This is because pregnant women are at increased risk of developing *symptomatic* urinary tract infections. This is a threat not only to the mother but also to the developing fetus. Thus, urine cultures are routinely obtained in caring for asymptomatic pregnant women.

The most important time to break Rule 5 is when you get vaccinated. Infectious diseases specialists are particularly aware of the extraordinary benefits of vaccines for healthy people. Here the goal is to keep you feeling well—that is, asymptomatic.

The remarkable impact of immunization is difficult to exaggerate. Currently, routine childhood vaccination protects against ten viral infections: measles, mumps, rubella (German measles), chickenpox, polio, two types of hepatitis, diarrhea, influenza, and (for girls) cancer of the cervix. Routine immunizations also provide protection against six bacterial infections: diphtheria, tetanus (lockjaw), pertussis (whooping cough), meningitis, pneumonia, and otitis media (middle ear infections).

Many of these infections remain scourges in the developing world, where vaccines are often unavailable. Measles is responsible for more than 150,000 deaths per year, mainly in children. Bacterial meningitis also claims more than 150,000 lives per year. Hepatitis B kills more than one million people per year. (To read more about immunization, see the appendix.)

In addition to recommending routine vaccinations for people with no symptoms, doctors sometimes recommend treatments based only on signs of disease (i.e., abnormal findings on physical exam or laboratory tests). When the evidence is clear that treatment is beneficial—if, for example, you have high blood pressure or a high blood cholesterol level—then breaking Rule 5 is often a good idea. However, always make sure you understand your doctor's reasoning. Shared decision making calls for a discussion with your doctor about the evidence, especially if you feel well.

Never Trust Anyone Completely, Especially Purveyors of Conventional Wisdom

P hillip Peterson, a 65-year-old American physician, developed shaking chills while standing at a hotel registration desk in Bangkok. The shaking was so violent that his wife thought he was having a seizure. Phil and his wife had just finished two weeks of travel in Vietnam and Thailand with two friends and had arrived that afternoon in Bangkok. They would fly back to the United States the next morning.

Except for thyroid hormone, which he had been taking for seven years, Phil wasn't taking any medicines. His health had been excellent most of his life, and until now he had not been sick during this trip.

When he entered the hotel room, he immediately turned off the air conditioner and asked his wife to call for more blankets. As soon as they arrived, he piled them on.

Before the trip, Phil had visited the Centers for Disease Control and Prevention (CDC) website for advice to travelers. Based on its advice, he didn't take any drugs to prevent malaria.

Because he is an infectious diseases specialist, he had a mental list of potential causes of fever in travelers to tropical countries. But he was surprised that he didn't have any symptoms other than feverishness and intense chills. He had no headache, muscle pains, nausea, vomiting, diarrhea, cough, sore throat, or runny nose.

Phil called the hotel's house doctor. Despite the absence of any symptoms to suggest a respiratory tract infection, he was told over the phone that "you have a cold."

Knowing that the house doctor's diagnosis was wrong, Phil called an infectious diseases colleague in Chiang Mai. They discussed several possible diagnoses, such as malaria, typhoid fever, and dengue. Meanwhile, Phil was thinking of Rule 6: Never trust anyone completely, especially purveyors of conventional wisdom. Had the CDC misled him? Did he indeed have malaria?

His colleague in Chiang Mai thought dengue was more likely, but the absence of any symptoms other than a fever and chills was unusual. He suggested waiting two hours to see whether other symptoms developed.

As it turned out, both doctors were wrong.

As Phil lay shivering under the covers, he mentally reviewed his medical history. He remembered having the same problem (feverishness and severe chills, but no other symptoms) ten years earlier, after eating pumpkin seeds one Thanksgiving morning. The episode cleared within three hours, just in time for him to join his family for dinner.

And pumpkin seeds had been served as a snack on the flight to Bangkok.

When Phil's colleague called back, they agreed that an allergy to something in pumpkin seeds was the most likely cause of his fever. Two hours later his fever broke, and he flew home the next morning with his much-relieved wife and their friends. He has carefully avoided pumpkin seeds since then.

> **Always doubt what you believe.**
>
> Epictetus (ca. 55–135)

As described in this (my) case, fever was the main symptom. When I examined myself, I felt hot to the touch. I didn't need a thermometer to know my temperature was elevated, and I guessed it was at least 103 degrees. When the hotel's doctor ascribed my fever to a cold, I knew he couldn't be trusted. After all, I didn't have any of the other symptoms that go along with an upper respiratory tract infection.

I was sure my colleague in Chiang Mai was more knowledgeable than I am about the causes of fever in Thailand. However, both of us were skeptical about dengue as the cause of my fever, because I didn't have any of the other symptoms associated with this viral infection. (To read about fever in general, and about dengue in particular, see the appendix.) I also questioned the conventional wisdom of the CDC; I thought maybe I should have taken a medication to prevent malaria. Yet I didn't have any of the other symptoms associated with malaria, such as a headache, muscle pain, fatigue, or diarrhea.

RULE
6

As demonstrated by my case, skepticism is hugely important for doctors. When caring for patients, they need to question even their own judgment. And you, the patient, also need to question your doctor if a recommendation is made that doesn't make sense to you.

In clinical education, the main purveyors of conventional wisdom are attending physicians. These are the doctors who supervise and teach students and residents about the care of patients. For these physicians, Rule 6 warns against overreliance on their personal experience. They don't purposely distort the truth. They just tend to forget that new evidence is constantly emerging that may challenge their set way of thinking. For trainees and for patients, Rule 6 underscores the importance of being wary about blindly accepting conventional wisdom.

Skepticism on the part of doctors is especially important whenever a new drug or treatment is promoted as being superior to older treatments. Even evidence-based medicine, founded on randomized clinical trials, must be viewed with skepticism until sufficient experience is gained. It takes time for the true merits and dangers to be fully appreciated.

As a rule, the medical literature is biased in favor of new and improved treatments. However, it is not uncommon for a treatment that initially makes good scientific sense—and is supported by early clinical trials—to be discredited by later clinical studies.

Trust is *the* cornerstone of the doctor-patient relationship. First and foremost, your doctor should trust you. This is why you *must* provide your doctor with an accurate accounting of your illness and concerns. Don't let your fear of an underlying disease (such as cancer) cloud the story you tell your doctor. When discussing your alcohol use, don't underestimate how much you drink. Ditto for smoking. Similarly, be sure to disclose any unsafe sex or use of illegal drugs. If you don't, you may lead your doctor down the wrong diagnostic path. Honesty could save your life.

Applying Rule 6

> Trust your instinct to the end, though you can render no reason.
>
> Ralph Waldo Emerson (1803–1882)

Trust in your physician is essential. You need to trust that any doctor who cares for you is well trained, keeps abreast of important developments, will do everything necessary to keep you healthy, and, when you are sick, will do everything possible to restore you to good health.

But how do you know whether you can trust your doctor's recommendations? As with all the Rules, common sense should be your guide. *If what your doctor recommends doesn't make sense to you, it probably isn't sensible.*

Explain to your doctor why a recommendation doesn't make sense to you, and ask your doctor to set you straight. Ask why he or she is making that recommendation. If it still doesn't make sense, get another medical opinion, or another doctor. In fact, as a general principle, *if you don't trust your doctor, get a different one.*

It was clear to me that the hotel's doctor in Bangkok couldn't be trusted, so I called my colleague in Chiang Mai for another opinion. Based on my symptoms of fever and shaking chills, he offered some potential diagnoses—but he was wise enough not to trust those diagnoses, because he had limited information. He wisely called back later to see whether I had developed any additional symptoms.

> Be careful what you read; it could kill you.
>
> **Anonymous**

In my case, before embarking on my trip, I had accessed the CDC's Travelers' Health website—an authoritative resource for travelers to countries such as Vietnam and Thailand. I was surprised to find that malaria wasn't listed as a risk in the areas I would be visiting. When I developed a fever, however, I thought to myself, Can't even the CDC be trusted?

The Internet has become the go-to source for information on virtually everything, including health-related issues. How trustworthy this information is generally corresponds to the quality of the site providing it. The Mayo Clinic, the National Institutes of Health (Health Information), and WebMD all have credible websites that provide valuable information on many medical problems. Cautious reading of their online material can serve as a useful supplement to the information you get from your doctor.

More than a century ago, Sir William Osler gave this warning: "A physician who treats himself has a fool for a patient."

Doctors need to be especially careful not to trust themselves to diagnose and treat their own illnesses.

A few years ago, I began to manifest the symptoms of hyperthyroidism. I lost 10 pounds in two weeks and was so short of breath I could barely walk up a flight of stairs. My wife, an attorney, detected my rapid pulse—a sign of hyperthyroidism. She urged me to see a doctor. I rudely reminded her that I didn't tell her how to practice law. After two weeks of refusing to listen, I finally saw my internist, who quickly diagnosed my problem as an overactive thyroid. The lesson here: trust your loved ones.

Rule 6 is particularly useful in guiding nonmedical decisions. The purveyors of conventional wisdom—professors, political pundits, public policy wonks, economists, meteorologists—are best viewed with a healthy degree of skepticism.

Breaking Rule 6

If you have a doctor you trust—one whose recommendations make sense to you—you can break Rule 6. The same can be said for authoritative, trustworthy online resources. For example, I was happy to learn that the CDC's Travelers' Health website (wwwnc.cdc.gov/travel) can be trusted. Another web-based resource, the Cochrane Library (http://cochrane.org/reviews), can be trusted for recommendations on treatment. The Cochrane Library doesn't cover all medical disorders, but the treatments for a large number of conditions are subjected to thorough, nonbiased, evidence-based review.

Most Things Are What They Seem to Be, Except When They're Not

Roberto Sanchez was an 18-year-old star high school athlete—captain of the football team. He played basketball and lifted weights. Since graduation he had been working in a lumber yard. When he was admitted to our hospital several months after graduation, he couldn't walk up a flight of steps because of fatigue and difficulty breathing.

Roberto described his other symptoms: for the past two weeks he had felt feverish and had been awakened by night sweats. The doctor who examined him in our emergency room noticed a tenderness in the right side of his abdomen, over his liver. She also noticed that the whites of his eyes were yellow. The admitting diagnosis was viral hepatitis.

That evening, when medical residents examined Roberto, they confirmed that his liver was tender and his eyes were yellow. He also had a fever—his temperature was 102.4 degrees. Like the ER doctor, the residents thought Roberto had viral hepatitis. Test results showing abnormal liver function supported this idea.

The next morning, however, his doctors shifted their attention from Roberto's liver to his heart. He was now short of breath while lying in bed, and when a doctor examined his lungs with a stethoscope, she heard a crackly sound. Roberto's heart was failing.

A cardiologist was called in. He noticed a heart murmur that had been ignored in the ER and by the admitting doctors.

Later that afternoon I was asked to see Roberto. By that time, it was clear that Roberto's case fit Rule 7: Most things are what they seem to be, except when they're not. This wasn't viral hepatitis. Roberto's liver was tender, results from his liver function tests were abnormal, and his eyes were yellow—all because his liver was congested with blood from his failing heart.

Results of cultures of blood samples taken in the ER established the diagnosis. Roberto had an infection of one of the valves of his heart, caused by a bacterium called *Haemophilus influenzae*. I recommended antibiotics appropriate for this infection. When I examined him, I, too, noted a heart murmur caused by failure of his mitral valve.

Roberto was transferred to our cardiac intensive care unit for close observation. I thought that this probably wasn't necessary, since he was a strapping, otherwise healthy 18-year-old. Also, I thought an infection of the mitral valve wasn't as serious as an infection of the aortic valve.

When I came to the hospital the next morning, I learned that in the middle of the night, Roberto had developed full-blown heart failure. He was taken to the operating room for emergency valve replacement. He didn't survive the surgery.

For many months after Roberto's death, the doctors involved in his care discussed how to prevent such a tragic outcome in the future.

Donald Petree was a 32-year-old businessman whom I saw in the infectious diseases clinic. His chief symptom was three weeks of fever. His only other symptom was feeling unusually tired. He had been evaluated by his primary care physician eight days earlier. Because his white blood cell count showed an increased number of cells called lymphocytes, Donald's doctor had ordered a test for infectious mononucleosis. The result was negative.

When I saw Donald, his temperature was 101.2. I examined his neck and found several swollen lymph glands. Donald told me he had been married for five years and had a healthy 3-year-old son who attended day care. Although Donald's family life was happy, he told me that he'd had unprotected sex with a prostitute during a business trip two months earlier.

I ordered another blood count. Once again it showed an increased number of lymphocytes, some with an atypical appearance. When I reviewed the blood film with a pathologist, we agreed that the findings were most consistent with a viral infection: infectious mononucleosis, cytomegalovirus (CMV) infection, or infection with the AIDS virus (HIV). Because Donald's test for infectious mononucleosis had proved negative and he reported unprotected sex with a prostitute,

I feared an HIV infection. Certainly, such an infection was possible, if not likely.

I shared my concern with Donald. I told him that because it was Friday afternoon, I wouldn't have the HIV or other lab results back until Monday. In the meantime, I told him to try not to worry, though I did counsel him not to have sexual relations with his wife until we had established the diagnosis.

On Monday morning I was reminded of Rule 7: Most things are what they seem to be, except when they're not. I was relieved to learn that Donald's HIV test result was negative, and the results of the test for CMV pointed to an acute CMV infection. I called him to share this good news. I also told him that although I couldn't say for sure, he may have acquired this viral infection from his son, as children often pick up CMV infections in day care. And I told him his CMV infection would almost certainly get better on its own.

Donald was greatly relieved by this news. Then he told me he hadn't slept all weekend. He had even considered suicide over the thought of having to tell his wife about a diagnosis of HIV.

I apologized for raising the possibility of HIV infection before the test results were in. I had been right to tell him not to worry, but wrong in suggesting a possible diagnosis that was logical but unestablished.

> We see only what we know.
> Johann Wolfgang von Goethe (1749–1832)

Although I have difficulty remembering phone numbers and the names of new acquaintances, the memories of the mistakes I have made in caring for patients are as vivid as those of the days my children were born. And flashbacks of the anguish in cases like Roberto Sanchez's continue to haunt me. I suspect the same is true for all doctors. Most of these mistakes hinge upon Rule 7: Most things are what they seem to be, except when they're not.

In Roberto's case, a mistaken impression by the ER physician that he had viral hepatitis biased the thinking of other doctors. This error, a type that Jerome Groopman, in *How Doctors Think*, refers to as "diagnosis momentum," diverted attention from Roberto's heart, which was failing to pump blood efficiently. His mitral valve was falling apart because of a bacterial infection. This infection, called endocarditis, is one of the most serious of all infections. Without antibiotic treatment, it is always fatal. (To read more about endocarditis, see the appendix.)

When I saw Donald Petree in the infectious diseases clinic, I thought I was an expert on CMV disease. By that time, I had spent most of my career studying the havoc this virus causes in patients who have a compromised immune system. But as Goethe observed, we see only what we know. Donald's immune system was normal. And I knew HIV caused a clinical picture just like his. But that didn't mean he had HIV. If I had been more aware of the potential role that day care centers play in the spread of CMV, I would have kept quiet about HIV until the results of his blood tests were back. (To find

RULE
7

out more about CMV infections and infections in day care centers, see the appendix.)

One of the many rewards of being a physician is the opportunity to learn something new every day. I hate mentioning this to medical students, however, as they are just beginning to learn the seemingly infinite nuances of diseases.

Rarely do patients have all of the symptoms and signs of a disease as described in medical textbooks. Dealing with this extraordinary complexity is one of medical professionals' major challenges.

Applying Rule 7

> **The only real mistake is the one from which we learn nothing.**
> John Powell (1963–)

The mistakes your doctor makes can benefit you, as long as he or she has learned from them. I learned a great deal from my mistakes in Roberto's and Donald's cases, and I plan to never repeat them. Paradoxically, however, it's because experience is such an important teacher that I make these recommendations:

- You need a doctor who has learned from his or her errors.
- You need a doctor who is forthright about his or her mistakes.
- You need a doctor whose mistakes weren't medical malpractice.

Because we all make mistakes, you don't want a doctor who thinks he or she is always right. If your doctor is defensive or arrogant when questioned about an unexpected bad outcome, think about finding another doctor.

There is no practical way to find out about the number or kinds of mistakes your doctor has made. And it is difficult—if not impossible—to know whether the doctor learned from them. But you don't want a doctor whose mistakes resulted in malpractice (a topic discussed in connection with Rule 8).

My wife's recent experience provides an example of how to apply Rule 7. She noticed increasing trouble with double vision, but only at night and usually after spending many hours reading. When she told me of this, I immediately referred her to an ophthalmologist. After examining her, the eye specialist suggested that she might have a serious disease called myasthenia gravis.

Without asking for any further information from me, my wife read about myasthenia gravis on the Internet and concluded that this diagnosis made no sense. She decided against the diagnostic tests recommended by the ophthalmologist and, instead, went straight to an experienced neurologist. His diagnosis: age-related double vision caused by tired eye muscles. This made sense to her.

It turned out that she and the neurologist were right. Best of all, her condition was easily treated by wearing eyeglasses with prisms at night. My wife has lived with me long enough to know that all doctors make mistakes.

Everyone makes mistakes in their nonmedical decisions, of course. And as in most faulty medical decisions, hindsight

RULE
7

often makes these mistakes clear—sometimes very painfully so.

Breaking Rule 7

Most of the time, of course, things are precisely what they seem to be. Remember that adage in the discussion of Rule 4? In the United States, the sound of hoof beats usually does mean horses; in Kenya, the same sound usually means zebras. Doctors and patients alike need to remember that exceptions are real. Still, overemphasizing exceptions contributes to unnecessary anxiety, unnecessary tests, and medical costs.

For example, cancer is one possible cause of low back pain and headaches. However, the odds are overwhelming that if you develop either of these very common symptoms, it's not because of cancer. Your doctor shouldn't start with an expensive diagnostic procedure, such as a CT or MRI scan. Step one should be taking a thorough medical history and doing a physical exam.

And remember: if you don't agree with your doctor's advice, ask for a second medical opinion. Or do as my wife did on her own: find another doctor.

What Your Doctor Doesn't Know Could Kill You

Judging by the many family members and friends who visited the hospital when Pamela Ferguson died, she was greatly loved. Her death came as a shock to everyone. She was only 38 years old. Except for obesity, she enjoyed good health until two days before her hospitalization.

Pamela was an accountant who developed an irritating cough, sore throat, muscle pains, and fever. She felt so sick that she stayed home from work.

Her primary care doctor saw her the day before she was admitted to our hospital. He wasn't all that concerned about Pamela's symptoms. She told him that no one she knew was sick with a similar illness. She had not traveled outside Minnesota in the past two years. She had no exposure to animals. She did not smoke or drink alcohol. She was happily married, with two children, both under the age of 6.

The only abnormalities her primary care doctor found when he examined her were her weight (275 pounds) and a fever (temperature of 102.4 degrees). His evaluation of her lungs was difficult because of her weight, but he found no signs of pneumonia. He told her she had a viral infection and should go home, rest, and drink plenty of fluids.

Over the course of the next day, however, Pamela's breathing became progressively more difficult. When she called her doctor the next morning, he instructed her to go immediately to the emergency room. She could barely get out of bed, due to shortness of breath. Her husband called an ambulance, which brought her to our ER.

In the ER, all her vital signs were abnormal. Her blood pressure was low (90/40), and her pulse, respiratory rate, and temperature were all high. Her breathing was labored, and when the ER doctor examined her lungs with a stethoscope, she heard a diffuse crackly sound.

Pamela was given a dose of an antibiotic and taken immediately to the intensive care unit. A chest x-ray in the ICU showed a "white out"—abnormalities in both of her lungs that suggested severe pneumonia. She was promptly put on a respirator.

It was the fall of 2009, when a second wave of H1N1 influenza—swine flu—cases was mounting. Pamela's doctors thought she could have a severe H1N1 influenza virus infection. She was given the antiviral drug Tamiflu (oseltamivir). She was also treated with antibiotics to kill a potential bacterial infection that could cause life-threatening pneumonia.

The test results came back two days later. Pamela had H1N1 influenza.

Despite intensive management by the critical care staff and

input from our infectious diseases consultation service, Pamela's condition continued to deteriorate. After five days in the hospital, she was unresponsive. It had become impossible to support her breathing, due to severe viral pneumonia.

After difficult and painful discussions among the critical care physicians, Pamela's husband, and her parents, she was taken off the respirator. On the seventh day of her hospitalization, Pamela was pronounced dead.

All the doctors who had cared for Pamela shared her family's grief. And at some point, they all thought, What if her primary care doctor had started Tamiflu the day he saw her? All of them also reflected on Rule 8: What your doctor doesn't know could kill you.

> There are known knowns. These are things we know that we know. There are known unknowns. That is to say, there are things that we know we don't know. But there are also unknown unknowns. There are things we don't know we don't know.
>
> Donald Rumsfeld (1932–)

I wasn't the infectious diseases consultant in Pamela Ferguson's case. I learned of her tragic death several months later, from my colleagues.

It wasn't clear to us what viral infection her primary care doctor had in mind when he saw Pamela the day before she was hospitalized. If he was thinking of the flu, he had that right. But it is unlikely that he was thinking of H1N1 infection—the swine flu. If he had suspected an H1N1 infection and had started the antiviral drug Tamiflu a day earlier, it might have saved her life. But in October 2009, when Pamela came to him, this was one of the "unknown unknowns."

Nobody could fault Pamela's primary care doctor in 2009 for not prescribing Tamiflu. But now we know that obesity is a risk factor for developing severe or fatal H1N1 influenza. Today, a wise physician who examined an obese patient with suspected flu would prescribe Tamiflu, or a similar antiviral drug, immediately. (To read more about H1N1 influenza and other emerging infections, see the appendix.)

All medical schools in the United States regularly hold "morbidity and mortality conferences." The goal of these conferences is to improve the quality of patient care. Cases are presented of patients who suffered (morbidity) or died (mortality) as a result of medical errors.

The cases are usually presented as unknowns (that is, the final diagnosis is not revealed to the audience when the case is first presented). "Red herrings" (information that is not relevant to the case) are usually added, to throw the students, residents, and experts—the teaching faculty—off the trail to the right diagnosis. When the final diagnosis is disclosed, it often turns out that none of the experts had it right.

The main purpose, however, is not to stump the experts. Rather, it is to educate doctors so they will avoid similar errors in their own medical practices.

Occasionally, these errors aren't the honest mistakes that all practitioners make, but are mistakes that represent medical malpractice—a deviation from the accepted standard of care resulting in undue injury to a patient. Malpractice is not common, but it is quite real.

About half of all physicians, regardless of their ability, are sued for malpractice at least once during their careers. A large percentage of these suits are dismissed or found to have no merit. Nonetheless, they cause enormous emotional distress—for both patients and doctors. A much smaller percentage represent malpractice. The main factor underlying many malpractice lawsuits, however, is not a violation of the standard of care but a poor doctor-patient relationship.

Applying Rule 8

> None of us is as smart as all of us.
>
> Japanese proverb

When I was a medical student, the doctor who taught us how to take a patient's history was regarded as the leading internist at our school. It was rumored that when he was asked why he was so successful, he answered, "Because I get the best consulting doctors."

The critical importance of bringing in consulting physicians is supported by a study of infectious diseases malpractice cases that I conducted with three colleagues. We reviewed more than 150 malpractice suits settled by a large national malpractice insurance company. In not a single case did the doctor in charge request consultation by a specialist. In fact, the major recommendation we had at the end of the study was that doctors should seek help whenever they are faced with puzzling problems.

RULE
8

Thus, the best way for you to apply Rule 8 is to go to a primary care doctor who

- Is willing and able to get expert input from specialists when needed.
- Participates in ongoing training and continuing education.
- Has years or decades of experience.
- Actively engages you in decisions about tests and treatments.

Primary care doctors for adults are called general internists; for children, they are called pediatricians. When they care for patients of all ages, they may also be called practitioners of family medicine, general practice doctors, or doctors who practice combined medicine and pediatrics.

Following the passage of the Affordable Care Act in 2010, tens of millions of previously uninsured Americans will be looking for primary care doctors. Regardless of what people think about this particular effort at health care reform, the debate over the legislation does shine light on the importance of primary care. The challenge now is to develop strategies to address the shortage of primary care doctors, which is projected to reach between twenty-one and thirty thousand by 2015.

Finding a good doctor is often a complex process. Dozens of websites provide information on doctors, but these sites are far from perfect. In most cases, the information is very limited, outdated, or potentially biased. Don't rely heavily on these sites.

When you search for a doctor, look for the following information:

- *The doctor's resume (or curriculum vitae).* This document contains information about where and when the doctor trained, the doctor's areas of medical expertise, the honors and awards the doctor has received, and the doctor's certification by medical specialties.
- *State medical board data.* In the United States, state medical licensing agencies usually provide information on a physician's age, where the doctor went to medical school and completed residency training, whether the doctor's medical license is active, and certification by specialty and subspecialty organizations. In some states, a history of criminal convictions is given as well. (Certainly, any criminal conviction should raise a red flag.)

Unfortunately, finding information about physician malpractice is difficult, at best. And no sources of information will tell you whether a doctor obtains expert consultation when it is needed.

The best sources of information about doctors are other doctors. If you have a friend who is a physician or knows a physician, ask whom he or she would recommend. Other health care professionals—especially nurses and physician assistants—are also good sources of information about the doctors who can be trusted to take good care of you.

Life is full of risks. Applying Rule 8 to nonmedical decisions can help you avoid the really big mistakes—the ones

RULE
8

that can kill you. For example, when traveling abroad, the biggest risk to your health is not infections or other diseases but traffic accidents. When you rent a car, drive defensively. And when you can choose among taking a train, a bus, or a car, opt for the train.

Breaking Rule 8

A good example of when Rule 8 needs to be broken involves the timing of treatment of bacterial meningitis, a life-threatening infection. In my early years as an infectious diseases consultant, I followed the guidelines of the authorities who recommended holding off on antibiotic therapy until the results of certain diagnostic tests were known. But later studies showed that it is actually more important *not* to delay treatment. Thus, the guideline changed to giving antibiotics immediately, based only on the patient's symptoms (headache, fever, and confusion) and a physical sign (a stiff neck). It became clear that in such cases, it is better not to compromise a patient's chances of survival by worrying about getting laboratory tests before starting treatment. The doctors who did *not* adhere to Rule 8 in the old days turned out to be right. Their immediate administration of an antibiotic—because they suspected, although did not know for sure, that the patient had meningitis—saved the lives of many people. What the doctors did not know (in this case, whether the patient definitively had bacterial meningitis) could have killed their patients only if they failed to order an antibiotic before the diagnosis was established.

Timing Is Everything, and Sometimes Time Is the Cure

Paul Kreitzler, a 43-year-old musician, was admitted to our hospital complaining of two days of severe lower back pain, fever, and shaking chills. He was known to have metastatic cancer of the anus, diagnosed five months earlier. Also, for the past year he had been taking a combination of antiviral drugs, called highly active antiretroviral therapy (HAART), for an HIV infection. He had contracted HIV ten years earlier, when he had unsafe sex with an infected partner.

When he was admitted to our hospital, Paul's temperature was 102.8 degrees. He was writhing in pain, which was localized in his lower back. An examination of his back didn't reveal any signs of tenderness, swelling, or redness, and when a physician examined his abdomen, she found no signs of a perforated intestine. Initial laboratory studies showed a markedly elevated white blood cell count. X-rays of his chest, abdomen, and back revealed no abnormalities.

Considering Paul's symptoms and the high white blood

cell count, his doctors suspected an acute bacterial infection. A combination of antibiotics active against a variety of bacteria was started immediately.

The next day, the blood culture results came back positive for *Escherichia coli* (better known simply as *E. coli*), a bacterium normally found in the gastrointestinal tract. This microbe is also the most common cause of urinary tract infections. After the urine culture came back as negative, however, Paul's bowel seemed the most likely source of his *E. coli* bloodstream infection. Because the spread of his anal cancer involved multiple areas of the bowel, the cancer seemed to play a role in the development of his bloodstream infection.

Although his temperature returned to normal within 48 hours of admission, Paul continued to complain of severe low back pain. His admitting doctor ordered a CT scan of his lower back. Paul's doctors were worried that his ongoing back pain could be due to an abscess, his cancer, or a herniated spinal disk. However, the CT scan result was normal.

Paul had been given morphine since he first arrived at the hospital, but it didn't completely relieve his pain. Nonetheless, he wanted to go home, where he could continue taking a strong painkiller and complete a course of antibiotics. Because he no longer had a fever and his white blood cell count had returned to almost normal, this seemed reasonable.

But, just before his discharge, the pain increased—and moved to his upper left thigh. When his doctor examined this area, she felt an unusual, sponge-like sensation. She ordered another CT scan, which revealed gas in the thigh tissue.

Suddenly, Paul's doctors realized that precious time

shouldn't be lost and that the first part of Rule 9, timing is everything, needed to be applied in spades. They suspected a life-threatening infection called necrotizing fasciitis, and they called in a surgeon.

The surgeon examined Paul and quickly took him to the operating room, where he removed a great deal of dead tissue from Paul's upper left leg.

Multiple surgeries to remove more dead tissue followed. Despite intensive surgical and medical treatment, Paul died ten days after he was first hospitalized.

> **The opportunity is often lost by deliberating.**
> **Publilius Syrus (85–43 BCE)**

Paul Kreitzler had battled HIV infection for at least ten years. His anal cancer, caused by another sexually transmitted virus—human papilloma virus (HPV)—had been a problem for months. While both of these viruses took a serious toll, it was a bacterial infection—necrotizing fasciitis—that quickly took Paul's life.

Paul's case illustrates the critical importance of the timing of treatment. Of his three fundamental principles of making smart health choices, described in *Decision Tree: Taking Control of Your Health in the New Era of Personalized Medicine*, Thomas Goetz prioritizes early treatment: "The first rule: early is better than late." From the dawn of antiviral therapy for HIV to this very day, clinical trials have tried to answer the question of when to start treatment. Nevertheless, if Paul had started HAART earlier, he might well be alive today. And

RULE
9

if the vaccine that prevents HPV infection had been available when he was a young man, his life might have been spared.

We do know with certainty, however, that the necrotizing fasciitis that killed Paul requires immediate surgical intervention. Paul's pain, localized at first in his lower back, puzzled everyone, but in retrospect, the severity of his pain pointed to the ultimate diagnosis. Unfortunately, by the time he developed gas in his thigh, it was too late.

Decisions about the proper timing of treatment involve both urgent situations, such as necrotizing fasciitis, and circumstances when doing nothing, called "watchful waiting"—applying the cure of time—is more beneficial. Although people who are infected with HIV rarely, if ever, get better on their own, they typically feel well for ten years or even longer. Once someone starts taking HAART, a drug cocktail that must be taken for life, the person is subjected to potential side effects and toxicity. Doctors want to protect their patients from this downside of therapy as long as possible.

Entities should not be multiplied beyond necessity.

William of Ockham (1285–1349)

Patients can have as many diseases as they damn well please.

John B. Hickman, M.D. (1914–1970)

Paul's case also points out the challenge of medical decision making for patients with diseases as complex as HIV infection. As a rule, our thinking is guided by Ockham's (or Occam's) Razor—a principle attributed to the medieval Franciscan friar William of Ockham. The principle says that if there are several hypotheses, it's best to choose the one that makes the fewest assumptions. Most of the time, doctors look for a single unifying diagnosis that ties together all of a patient's symptoms and signs. In other words, doctors like to keep things simple.

The counterargument to this notion is the principle espoused by the late Dr. John Hickham, former chairman of medicine at Indiana University Medical School. This notion, known as Hickham's Dictum, points out that patients can have more than one disease at a time.

Very few diseases are as complicated as HIV/AIDS. Hickham's Dictum often applies for people who have this disease, as it did in Paul's case. He suffered from HIV infection for years, but he died of an acute bacterial infection. Additionally, he developed anal cancer caused by HPV. (To read more about HIV and HPV, see the appendix.)

Applying Rule 9

The best timing of all is prevention: taking steps to avoid illness in the first place. The next best involves seeking medical help sooner rather than later. This means
- Practicing behaviors that prevent disease.
- Getting trustworthy medical advice early.

> A stitch in time saves nine.
>
> **Anonymous**

- Seeing your doctor promptly once you have symptoms that are more than minor.
- Going immediately to urgent care or the emergency room if your symptoms suggest a serious or life-threatening condition.

About 40 percent of all deaths in the United States result from people failing to prevent illness by following these simple do's and don'ts:

- DO exercise, practice safe sex, wash your hands frequently, make sure your immunizations are up to date, take your medicines as prescribed, and get a good primary care doctor.
- DON'T smoke, drink alcohol to excess, overeat, text while driving, or be reckless about sex or choosing a doctor.

When you are sick, you're mainly interested in getting prompt, trustworthy advice. Most of the time, your primary care doctor is your best resource for this advice. But some symptoms require immediate attention, such as the sudden onset of left-sided chest pain, the abrupt development of weakness of an extremity, slurred speech, or a seizure. If you develop any of these symptoms, call 911 immediately for an ambulance. Let the emergency room doctors determine what to do next.

Timing also can be critical in your nonmedical decisions. This point was driven home vividly for me when my son-in-law moved to another city hundreds of miles away, with my daughter and grandchildren. My wife and I were mad at him for two months—until a lightning bolt hit and a fire destroyed the home they had moved out of. The firemen said it was fortunate they weren't there, as they all would have been killed. Our son-in-law has been our hero ever since.

Breaking Rule 9

> The art of medicine consists in amusing the patient while nature cures the disease.
>
> Voltaire (1694–1778)

In Voltaire's day, evidence-based medicine was not refined, and few medical treatments worked. His suggestion that humor is the best medicine may have reflected his concerns about the dangers of medical remedies in general, and of surgery, of the times. But it may also have reflected his wisdom that nature cures many diseases—if a patient is willing to be patient. Today, however, we have many effective treatments, both medical and surgical. The question addressed by Rule 9 is when they should be applied.

Sometimes, the best option really is waiting for nature to cure you. Because Rule 9 applies both to this "watchful waiting" approach and to immediate intervention, Rule 9 should rarely be broken. However, at the end of someone's life, medical and surgical treatments may become futile. Then the art of medicine involves relieving the patient's pain and discomfort rather than either waiting passively or attempting a cure.

Caring Is Always
Important Medicine

When she called me, Dr. Allison McGowan had recently celebrated her forty-fifth birthday. I had lost contact with her for about ten years, so it was nice to hear her upbeat voice again. Sadly, however, I learned that she was still suffering from chronic fatigue syndrome (CFS). She wanted my opinion about a medication recently touted as a breakthrough for CFS.

I first got to know Allison in the early 1990s, when she was training in our internal medicine residency program. She was a star: bright, hardworking, and deeply committed to her patients. She also had a great sense of humor. After completing her residency, she did a fellowship in cardiology and joined a busy clinical practice in St. Paul, Minnesota. She loved her work. However, when she first became ill with CFS in 1997, she was forced to quit.

Like most people who have CFS, Allison first experienced symptoms that suggested an acute viral infection—fever, sore throat, headache, muscle and joint pains, and fatigue. Also, like nearly everyone who develops an acute viral infection, she took to bed. However, she found that bed rest didn't relieve her exhaustion. Her fatigue was decidedly different from the tiredness she had often experienced after being up all night caring for patients. This fatigue wasn't relieved at all by sleep. She felt just as exhausted when she woke up in the morning as when she went to bed. And, notably, the fatigue got markedly worse when she tried any kind of physical activity.

When I first saw Allison as a patient in our infectious diseases clinic in 1998, she could barely walk up a flight of stairs. Before she developed CFS, she had been an accomplished mountaineer and kayaker. Now, not only had she abandoned a clinical practice she loved, but she had given up all forms of exercise.

On top of dealing with disabling fatigue, she was exasperated with her primary care doctor, as well as with several consultants. They all seemed completely unsympathetic to her plight. Her primary care doctor believed the problem was in her head. He referred her to a psychiatrist, who agreed with Allison that her head was just fine.

On examining her, I didn't find any abnormalities. The results of a battery of laboratory tests were all normal. Because Allison's clinical picture fit the diagnosis of CFS, I entered Allison into our University of Minnesota CFS research program.

When Allison phoned some ten years later, around her forty-fifth birthday, I learned she had moved from Minnesota to a much gentler climate. Disabling fatigue, unrefreshing sleep, and difficulties with concentration remained her main symptoms. I mentioned that CFS research was progressing in many countries, but a beneficial medication had yet to be found.

Allison reiterated that her primary care doctor had provided little comfort. Quite the contrary, she said. "You know, Phil, the best thing I ever did for my chronic fatigue syndrome was to get a horse."

As with most of the patients in our CFS research program, Allison was helped just by knowing that I cared. I took her illness seriously, even though we didn't yet (and still don't) know its cause. In our phone call, we both agreed that nowadays, some doctors seem to have forgotten their main calling—caring for patients. At that moment, Allison brought to mind Rule 10: Caring is always important medicine.

The greatest mistake in the treatment of diseases is that there are physicians for the body and physicians for the soul, although the two cannot be separated.

Plato (424–348 BCE)

For the secret of the care of the patient is in caring for the patient.

Francis W. Peabody (1881–1927)

RULE
10

Like all third-year medical students, when I started my first hospital rotation I was terrified. Every morning, I found myself at the bedside of very sick, and sometimes dying, patients. Every night, I lay awake worrying about them. It was clear that in addition to wanting medicine to relieve their symptoms, they wanted a doctor they could trust to do everything possible to restore them to health. Fortunately, that kind of doctor—called an attending physician—was in charge of their care.

Attending physicians are experienced practitioners who are responsible for overseeing the care of patients and for teaching new doctors and medical students. They also serve as a role model for trainees.

Classes during the first two years of medical school prepared me well for understanding the science behind many of the diseases I encountered. However, I was totally unprepared for practicing the *art* of medicine. Unlike the science of medicine, the art of medicine can't be learned from textbooks or in the classroom.

Attending physicians practice both the science and the art of medicine.

The art of medicine has to do with emotions. The art of medicine requires empathy—the ability to understand what a patient is going through. And in addition to feeling sympathy or sorrow for a sick patient, the artful practitioner has compassion. He or she has a strong desire to alleviate patients' suffering. While a keen interest in the scientific basis of health and disease is necessary to be a good doctor, compassion continues to be what draws students to medical careers.

Recent studies suggest that the empathy of medical students begins to decline in the third year of medical school, the first year in which they are primarily involved in patient care. Several factors erode this fundamental aspect of medical practice. The first is having to keep up with a very rapidly growing knowledge base; this challenge can result in brain overload. Second is the complexity of caring for patients, especially those who are critically ill. Third is an overreliance on a rapidly developing and highly sophisticated technology. (Taking a patient's history and performing a careful physical examination, however, are still the mainstays of diagnosis.) Fourth is the commercialization of medicine, as demonstrated by the emergence of a health care industry over the past several decades. Some of these same factors also contribute to the burnout of physicians already in practice.

Medical students are told early in their training that the best way to build empathy and compassion is to be a patient oneself. Another is to witness the impact of the serious or fatal illness of a loved one. Although none of us would voluntarily sign up for these two assignments, inevitably these experiences will come along—and they will be instructive.

Dr. Allison McGowan knows in her bones what empathy and compassion are all about. Unfortunately, her experience with an uncaring primary care doctor is shared by many patients suffering from CFS. (To read more about CFS, see the appendix.)

The scientific advances of the first decade of the twenty-first century are astonishing. Some authorities believe that medicine is at the threshold of its biggest shake-up in history.

> Although scientific knowledge is available to all, there is a vast difference between the best and worst doctors, that difference representing the art of medicine.
>
> Sir David Weatherall (1933–)

The Internet, teleconferencing, and cell phones already have revolutionized access to information and the means of communication between physicians and patients and between physicians.

Also, we are on the cusp of personalized medicine. This means having all of your twenty-four thousand or so genes (called a personal genome) characterized to guide decisions based on your risks for certain diseases and your likely reactions to medications. Some experts suggest that an individual's personal genome will eventually be available as an app on cell phones. Some even suggest that it won't be long before your doctor can scan virtually every organ in your body with a cell-phone-like device. For an informative overview of how such digital advances are transforming modern medicine, read Eric Topol's book *The Creative Destruction of Medicine: How the Digital Revolution Will Create Better Health Care*.

Yet, even as medicine is witnessing a sea change in science and technology, one thing hasn't changed: the art of medicine. At the turn of the twenty-first century, the Institute of Medicine popularized the term "patient-centered care," focusing on understanding the needs of the individual patient and tailoring treatment that is specific for each patient. Although technology can sometimes distance patients from their doctors, when used carefully and properly, the new digital advances (genomics, proteomics, and so on) can optimize your health. As David Agus notes in his book *The End of Illness*, "It's one size fits *you, not all.*"

In a commentary in the *Journal of the American Medical Association* in May 2011, titled "Patient-Physician Communication: It's about Time," Drs. Wendy Levinson and Philip Pizzo conclude, "Science and technology have advanced enormously over the last decades, but ultimately the best medical care requires deep knowledge of science as well as the skills to communicate effectively with patients. If the medical profession wishes to maintain or perhaps regain trust and respect from the public, it must meet patients' needs with a renewed commitment to excellence in communication skills of physicians. It is time to make this commitment." Hear! Hear!

In the past two decades, an interdisciplinary field called integrative medicine has emerged. Integrative medicine grew out of a recognition that practitioners of alternative or complementary medicine can also contribute to the well-being of patients. Integrative medicine is defined as "the practice of medicine that reaffirms the importance of the relationship between the practitioner and patient, focuses on the whole person, is informed by evidence, and makes use of all appropriate therapeutic approaches, health care professionals and disciplines to achieve optimal health and healing." What sets integrative medicine apart from alternative and complementary medicine is its emphasis on evidence.

At least twenty-two evidence-based studies (or randomized clinical trials) have been carried out with patients who have CFS. Only two modalities, cognitive behavioral therapy and graded exercise therapy, were found to be effective, and then only for some patients. As for getting a horse—what is formally called equine-facilitated therapy—this approach hasn't yet been tested in a randomized clinical trial. Nonetheless, since Allison found this alternative approach helpful, I recommended that she apply Rule 2: If what you're doing seems to be working, think about continuing it.

Applying Rule 10

> What do we want, when we become patients? We want, first of all, to be understood and to understand. . . . We want, above all else, to believe the right things were done for all the right reasons, at the right place at the right time.
>
> Beth Kephart

How can you be sure your doctor cares? How can you know whether your doctor not only has deep knowledge of the *science* of medicine but also practices the *art* of medicine?

You won't find the answer to this question in the diplomas on your doctor's office wall. And it's unlikely that you can gather this crucial information from a resume or curriculum vitae. Like art in a broader sense, you will feel it or know it when you see it.

A major sign that your doctor cares is reflected by the quality—not necessarily the quantity—of time he or she spends with you.

You want a doctor who

- Demonstrates a high level of compassion when you are sick.
- Listens carefully to you and your loved ones.
- Asks if you have any questions or concerns.
- Communicates effectively by giving clear and understandable explanations.
- Puts you in the driver's seat in decisions about diagnostic tests and treatments.
- Is honest and humble.
- Always provides hope.

When my wife was pregnant with our first child, her obstetrician was a famous and highly sought-after doctor. He would spend no more than ten minutes with her at each prenatal visit. Then we moved to another city, and she needed a new obstetrician. This physician spent considerably more time with her during prenatal visits.

Thus I was surprised when she complained about the second obstetrician and lauded the first. I asked why. She told me that the first obstetrician gave her his undivided attention during the entire visit. He answered her questions and allayed her anxiety about the upcoming delivery. The second obstetrician simply talked a lot.

All doctors have a responsibility to care for their individual patients, and caring also motivates those who work to alleviate suffering caused by poverty, injustice, or natural disasters. And because our fate is inextricably connected to the health of the animal world and the environment, there are, thankfully, many excellent caretakers (and caregivers) in these non-medical fields as well.

Breaking Rule 10

Rule 10 is the only Rule of Internal Medicine that should never be broken.

The Participatory Art of Medicine

- -

> The practice of medicine is an art, based on science.
> Sir William Osler (1849–1919)

In this book, you've read about how doctors arrive at a diagnosis by listening to a patient describe his or her symptoms and looking for signs of disease on physical exam and in laboratory tests.

You've read about patients who had infections or other clinical disorders that illustrate the Ten Rules of Internal Medicine. These same Rules apply to decision making for all types of medical problems.

Most importantly, you've read about how common sense—the basis of all the Rules—should guide medical decisions.

You've also read about how, in this era of shared decision making, good communication is critical. Your doctor wants your help; the art of medicine is a two-way street. Get up in the driver's seat. Ask questions, express your ideas, and discuss your worries and concerns.

A recurring theme throughout this book is the differences among individual patients. No two patients with the same disease have exactly the same symptoms and signs. Similarly, communication must be shaped by the wishes of the individual patient.

Doctors want their patients to be empowered and motivated to share in decisions about their health. But the extent, timing, and technique of doctors' disclosure of the scientific facts and the prognosis about certain medical conditions—especially terminal diseases—must take into account the individual patient's wishes. Truth telling isn't a one-way act of doctors providing information. Patients need to express their feelings and ask questions of their doctors in a private setting. The patient's emotional well-being, social support, religious beliefs, cultural background—all need to be considered. This is one of the reasons that all patients need a primary care doctor who gets to know them and, when appropriate, also gets to know their family members and close friends.

> **Real knowledge is to know the extent of one's ignorance.**
> **Confucius (551–479 BCE)**

Another recurring theme throughout this book is that all doctors make mistakes. Often, a lack of knowledge is the basis for these mistakes. Hindsight makes this clear. Spectacular as the advancement of medicine has been in recent years, we doctors shouldn't underestimate our limitations.

Paradoxically, the more I learn about medical problems, the less I seem to know. Most of the doctors whom I hold in high regard say the same thing. Along with increased clinical experience comes the realization that many patients suffer from conditions with an unknown cause—what medical professionals call idiopathic disorders. And we learn that for many medical conditions, even those for which we know the cause, such as infectious agents, our understanding and treatment are often inadequate. But one thing all doctors know for certain: to care honestly and earnestly for every patient.

Sir William Osler, the father of internal medicine, had it right more than a century ago. Medicine is an art informed by science. The better the science, the better the art.

In recent years, medicine has been increasingly viewed as a participatory art. Through two-way communication, medical decisions are shared by physicians and patients. To advance knowledge, patients are often asked to participate in clinical research. And patients also advance medical science by serving as advocates for increased funding of medical research. All of these efforts have helped to improve medical science, advance the art of medicine, and improve doctors' caring for patients.

The Rules Revisited

I don't expect you to remember all ten of the Rules. But when you are making a medical decision for yourself or someone you care about, the list below may be useful as a quick reminder. This list will help you choose the Rule or Rules you need in a specific situation and provide a recap of the key thinking behind each Rule.

The Ten Rules of Internal Medicine

Rule 1: **If You Don't Know What You're Doing, Don't Do Anything**

If you, or a loved one, are sick or concerned about something on a physical exam or test, speak up.
- If your doctor advises doing nothing, ask why.
- Ask about the evidence for and against proceeding with the offered treatments.

- Ask about all other potential options. For each option, ask about its potential benefits and risks.

Rule 2: If What You're Doing Seems to Be Working, Think about Continuing It

If you are taking a medication and doing well, this is a good rule to follow. Nevertheless, some further guidelines:

- Ask your doctor why he or she recommends continuing a particular medication or treatment.
- Make sure you understand exactly how long the treatment or course of medication will need to be.
- Ask about all other potential options. For each option, ask about its potential benefits and risks.
- Before you stop taking any medication earlier than prescribed, speak with your doctor and make sure you understand the potential consequences.

Rule 3: If What You're Doing Doesn't Seem to Be Working, Think about Doing Something Else

If you, or a loved one, are being treated and your condition is not improving, or is getting worse,

- Ask your doctor whether another treatment might work better—and find out what all other possible options are.
- Ask for a second medical opinion from a doctor with expertise related to your specific problem.

Rule 4: Don't Agree to an Invasive Procedure without Understanding Why It's Needed—and without Getting a Second Opinion

All surgical and other invasive procedures carry risks. If such a procedure is recommended, ask these questions:

- Is this invasive strategy necessary? Why?
- Is this the best way to treat my condition? Why?
- Are there any noninvasive treatments? If so, how effective are they? What are the potential risks and side effects of each one?

If surgery or some other invasive procedure is, in fact, the best (or the only good) option, ask these questions, as well:

- How long will the procedure take?
- Where will it be done?
- What are the potential risks?
- How long will recovery take?
- What surgeon would you go to if you (or your mother, father, or child) needed this operation? Why?

Rule 5: If You Don't Have Symptoms, a Doctor Can't Make You Feel Better

When you have no symptoms and your doctor recommends a drug, procedure, or other treatment, ask these questions:

- What are the potential risks and side effects of this drug, procedure, or treatment?
- What do you believe will probably happen if I don't

take this drug, or receive this treatment, or undergo this procedure?

If your doctor recommends a test and you have no symptoms, ask these questions:

- Why is this test necessary?
- What might happen if we don't do this test?

Rule 6: Never Trust Anyone Completely, Especially Purveyors of Conventional Wisdom

Trust is the cornerstone of your relationship with your doctor. As with all the Rules, however, common sense should be your guide.

- If what your doctor recommends doesn't make sense to you, it probably isn't sensible.
- Explain to your doctor why it doesn't make sense to you, and ask the doctor whether he or she can set you straight. Ask why the doctor is making that recommendation. If it still doesn't make sense, get another medical opinion.
- If you don't trust your doctor, get a different one.

Rule 7: Most Things Are What They Seem to Be, Except When They're Not

Although all doctors make mistakes,

- You need a doctor who has learned from his or her errors.

- You need a doctor who is forthright about his or her mistakes.
- You need a doctor whose mistakes weren't medical malpractice.

Rule 8: What Your Doctor Doesn't Know Could Kill You

You need a primary care doctor who
- Is willing and able to get expert input from specialists when needed.
- Participates in ongoing training and continuing education.
- Has years or decades of experience.
- Actively engages you in decisions about tests and treatments.

Rule 9: Timing Is Everything, and Sometimes Time Is the Cure

Because early treatment is advisable and because prevention is best, you should
- Practice behaviors that prevent disease.
- Get trustworthy medical advice early.
- See your doctor promptly if you have symptoms that are more than minor.
- Go immediately to urgent care or the emergency room if your symptoms suggest a serious or life-threatening condition.

RECAP

Rule 10: Caring Is Always Important Medicine

You need a primary care doctor who

- Demonstrates a high level of compassion when you are sick.
- Listens carefully to you and your loved ones.
- Asks whether you have any questions or concerns.
- Communicates effectively by giving clear and understandable explanations.
- Puts you in the driver's seat in decisions about diagnostic tests and treatments.
- Is honest and humble.
- Always provides hope.

Acknowledgments

This book wouldn't have come about if it weren't for three kinds of people: generators (health care professionals and patients who helped create the Rules), facilitators (experts who helped with the writing), and tolerators (family members who put up with this project).

Two of my infectious diseases colleagues were crucial in the development of the Rules. L. D. Sabath, head of the Infectious Diseases Division in the Department of Medicine at the University of Minnesota when I did my fellowship, taught me early versions of Rules 1 to 5. As I recall, he credited one of his mentors at Bellevue Hospital in New York City with their creation. David Williams, an infectious diseases colleague and close friend since 1975, encouraged me to publish the Ten Rules. And many medical students, residents, and patients contributed to all the Rules.

When I began writing this book, I thought I knew how to write nonfiction. After all, I had published many scientific papers throughout my medical career. But I learned that when it came to writing a book aimed at nonmedical readers, I knew almost nothing. Fortunately, I was steered to two great teachers. Scott Edelstein provided constructive criticism of four drafts of this book. I was amazed how consistently he improved my writing. Patricia Francisco—who, like Scott, teaches creative writing—also read many drafts of this book. Both saw merit in the project and encouraged me along the way. While both Scott and Patricia provided sage advice on the technical aspects of writing, they also get credit for helping me get inside the nonmedical reader's head.

I am also greatly indebted to Jackie Wehmueller, executive editor at the Johns Hopkins University Press, who not only contributed to the writing but saw the book through the publishing process. I also thank the copy editor, Linda Strange.

And finally, the tolerators—my wife, Karin, and my two children, Kirstin and Per—put up with hearing the Rules on innumerable occasions over the years. I thank them for their patience—and for providing many opportunities to adapt and use the Rules in making nonmedical decisions.

Appendix

Additional Information about the Common Illnesses Discussed in This Book

Topics Discussed in Rule 1
Encephalitis

> Compared to other infectious diseases, encephalitis has a high mortality. . . . It is hard to comprehend in this era of modern medicine that an infection can result in death.
>
> Elaine Dowell and Ava Easton, Encephalitis Society

Inflammation of the brain, also known as encephalitis, is one of the most frightening of all diseases. In the United States, encephalitis results in more than 19,000 hospitalizations and more than 1,400 deaths each year. In Southeast Asia, at least 65,000 people die of encephalitis caused by rabies virus or Japanese encephalitis virus every year. Although there is a vaccine that can prevent rabies if it is given shortly after exposure to the virus, for those who are vaccinated too late or not at all, rabies is a death sentence. Only a single case has been documented of a person with rabies encephalitis who survived the infection. The cause of encephalitis is often unknown. In fact, even using the most sophisticated diagnostic tests available, a cause cannot be found for more than half of encephalitis cases.

The now infamous West Nile virus was first described in 1937 in Egypt—thus the origin of its name. West Nile virus, however, did not make its way to the United States until 1999. The first cases were seen in the New York City area, in birds and then in humans. Subsequently, West Nile virus spread across the country via birds and mosquitoes and became the most common cause of encephalitis in the United States.

Most people who are bitten by a mosquito carrying the virus have no symptoms. Some have only a fever. But people over age 70 have an increased risk of developing a brain infection (known as viral encephalitis) after being bitten by an infected mosquito. It is also older people who suffer most of the serious complications and are more likely to die of the disease. Exactly why this is so is not well understood, but it is why older adults should liberally use mosquito spray from spring through early fall. There is no specific antiviral treatment for a person with this infection.

In addition to carrying West Nile virus, mosquitoes can transmit a host of other viruses (such as Western equine encephalitis virus, Eastern equine encephalitis virus, St. Louis encephalitis virus, and Lacrosse encephalitis virus). These can infect the brain itself (in which case the disease is called encephalitis) or the covering of the brain (in which case the disease is called meningitis).

Recently, Powassan virus has emerged as a cause of encephalitis in Canada and the United States. This virus is transmitted not by mosquitoes but by ticks. The deer tick, also known as the blacklegged tick, is particularly problematic, because this tick species can also harbor the bacterium that causes Lyme disease.

All the more reason to use a bug spray containing DEET, which keeps ticks and mosquitoes away.

Topics Discussed in Rule 2
Infections in People Who Have Had an Organ Transplant

> **Whether you're awaiting a kidney transplant or had your transplant long ago . . . the first step is learning as much as you can.**
>
> Chris Klug, www.transplantexperience.com

In 1954, the first kidney transplants from living donors to patients with end-stage kidney disease were performed. Over the decades that followed, hundreds of thousands of patients received transplanted kidneys, lungs, livers, pancreases, and intestines. Hundreds of thousands received bone marrow or stem cell transplants. And most recently, people have received transplanted faces.

In the early years of organ and bone marrow transplantation, opportunistic infections killed a large majority of transplant recipients. These infections take advantage of an immune system weakened by the drugs taken after the transplant procedure to depress the immune system so that it doesn't actively reject the transplanted organ. Today, with increased experience and improved immunosuppressive drugs, infections take much less of a toll. Currently, a large majority of people receiving transplants do remarkably well. The antibiotic trimethoprim-sulfamethoxisole prevents not only bacterial infections (nocardiosis, Legionnaires' disease, and listeriosis) but also a fungal infection (pneumocystosis).

In the early years of organ and bone marrow transplantation, cytomegalovirus (CMV) was by far the most common cause of infection in transplant recipients. Initially, it was unclear where the virus came from. But studies from many transplant centers showed that CMV, which lies dormant in many adults, reactivates when patients are given immunosuppressive drugs. An active infection can happen when the virus is harbored within the patient *or* when it is harbored in a transplanted organ, transplanted bone marrow, or transfused blood. Nowadays, methods for preventing CMV infection in transplant recipients are routine in developed countries. But new challenges, such as the management of infections in patients who travel to developing countries to receive transplants (so-called transplant tourists), continue to arise.

Topics Discussed in Rule 3
Methicillin-Resistant Staphylococcus aureus

> The head of the federal Centers for Disease Control and Prevention calls MRSA the "cockroach of bacteria." It's omnipresent, tough and adaptable.
>
> Carol Ostrom, *Seattle Times*

Even before methicillin-resistant *Staphylococcus aureus* (MRSA) came along, *Staphylococcus aureus* was the most dreaded of all bacterial species. This bacterium can cause life-threatening infections in healthy people. In addition to joint and bloodstream infections, other common sites of infection are the skin (cellulitis or boils), bones (osteomyelitis), lungs (pneumonia), and heart valves (endocarditis). In the 1980s, a toxin-producing *Staphylococcus au-*

reus strain swept the country, creating the epidemic of toxic shock syndrome.

When I finished my infectious diseases training in 1977, MRSA infections were a rarity in the United States. Only a few hospitals reported problems with MRSA in their burn units or intensive care units. By the late 1980s, however, a majority of *Staphylococcus aureus* infections in hospitals were due to hospital-associated MRSA (HA-MRSA). Except for infections in intravenous drug users in localized areas of the country, MRSA was never acquired outside the hospital.

All of this changed in 1997, when MRSA began spreading through the general community. Community-associated MRSA (CA-MRSA) rapidly became epidemic throughout the United States as well as other areas of the world.

Unlike HA-MRSA, CA-MRSA has captured widespread attention as the so-called superbug. No doubt this is in part due to the early years of the epidemic, when healthy children were its main victims. These CA-MRSA infections were often fatal.

Currently, in many areas of the United States, most *Staphylococcus aureus* infections acquired in the community are due to CA-MRSA. Not only is CA-MRSA resistant to many antibiotics, but it is also more virulent—that is, it causes much greater damage and a higher mortality than *Staphylococcus aureus* strains that are sensitive to methicillin.

In recent years, the rate of *Staphylococcus aureus* infections has declined, both in and outside hospitals. While doctors would like to believe this is due to better infection-control measures—such as frequent and thorough hand washing—the reason for this encouraging development is not yet understood.

A similar scenario was seen in the 1980s, when staphylococcal toxic syndrome seemed to emerge out of nowhere. Although tampon use was shown to be a major risk factor, it was unclear whether the decline of this life-threatening disease in the 1990s was related solely to a change in menstrual products. We still have much to learn about why certain infections arise and subside.

Topics Discussed in Rule 4
Tuberculosis

> More than two billion people, equal to one-third of the world's population, are infected with TB bacilli.
>
> **World Health Organization**

Tuberculosis (TB) is an infection that starts in the lungs. It is acquired by inhaling the tubercle bacterium coughed up by someone who is infected.

This bacterium has an unusual life cycle. Most of the time, it doesn't cause any symptoms when a person becomes infected; instead, it lies dormant in the body. This dormant form of TB, called latent TB, is the kind of infection that, if we tested every person on the planet, we'd find it in one of every three of them.

If a person's immune system becomes compromised at any time after the initial infection, the TB bacillus can awaken and reactivate. This is the case in most immigrants who develop TB. It is thought that the psychological stress associated with immigration suppresses the immune system and allows the bacillus to reactivate.

Antibiotics to treat TB were developed in the 1940s and 1950s.

Since then, the number of active TB cases in developed countries has decreased dramatically, but the disease hasn't been eradicated. In fact, more than nine million people are infected each year, resulting in more than one million deaths, primarily in the developing world where treatment isn't readily available.

In eighteenth-century Europe, TB was called the white plague. Much like bubonic plague (or the black death), which swept through Europe in the fourteenth century, killing 30 to 60 percent of the population, TB was the cause of death for one in three Europeans in the eighteenth century. When an antibiotic became available to treat TB in the mid-twentieth century, this was a colossal breakthrough. But the tubercle bacillus is a clever microbe. Doctors soon realized that they needed to administer more than one antibiotic at a time, to prevent a person from developing resistance to any of the antibiotics.

Today, infection by tubercle bacilli that are resistant to the two otherwise most-effective antibiotics is a worldwide problem called multi-drug-resistant TB, or MDRTB. Most worrisome is the emergence of an extremely drug-resistant strain of TB, called XDR-TB, which is resistant to almost all antibiotics. As of 2012, seventy-seven countries had confirmed cases of XDR-TB. Because untreated TB kills almost half the people it infects, a widespread XDR-TB outbreak would be like returning to the pre-antibiotic era.

Typhoid Fever

Typhoid fever is rare in the United States (fewer than 500 cases per year) but common in developing countries (between 12 and 33 million cases per year), where typhoid kills more than 200,000 people annually. Thus, typhoid fever is identified by the World Health Organization as a serious public health problem.

Poor hygiene is the underlying cause of the spread of typhoid fever. *Salmonella typhi*, the bacterium that causes typhoid fever, is transmitted by water or food contaminated with human feces. Public education campaigns encouraging people to wash their hands after defecating and before handling food are critical in controlling the spread of typhoid fever. Chlorination of drinking water, which kills *Salmonella typhi*, is thought to be responsible for the dramatic decrease of typhoid in the United States.

About a third of patients with untreated typhoid fever die. Antibiotic treatment reduces mortality to about 1 percent. But here, too, antibiotic resistance is emerging in many areas of the developing world. And if a splenic abscess develops, death is almost certain if the spleen isn't surgically removed.

About 5 percent of people who contract typhoid fever will continue to carry the typhoid bacillus after they recover. Such asymptomatic carriers are prohibited from working as food handlers. The infamous asymptomatic carrier Mary Mallon ("Typhoid Mary"), a young cook in early twentieth-century New York City, infected at least fifty-three people, three of whom died of the disease.

Traveling to a developing country where typhoid fever is common puts you at risk if you eat food prepared nonhygienically or drink water that isn't safe. However, a vaccine is available. If you are planning such a trip, consult your doctor or get advice at a travel clinic before you go, to see whether a typhoid vaccination is a good idea.

Topics Discussed in Rule 5
Urinary Tract Infections

> Urinary tract infections (UTIs) are considered to be the most common bacterial infection. Financially, the estimated annual cost of community-acquired UTI is significant, at approximately $1.6 billion.
> Betsy Foxman, University of Michigan School of Public Health

Studies carried out more than half a century ago demonstrated that it is abnormal to have many bacteria in our urine. However, in the 1970s, clinical research showed that treating urinary tract infections with antibiotics in adults with no symptoms provides no benefit. Furthermore, there is the risk of side effects of antibiotics, such as a life-threatening allergy.

Urinary tract infections are very common. As common infections go, they are second only to the common cold. More than four million doctor's office visits each year are for urinary tract infections.

Symptoms of a urinary tract infection include frequent urination, burning or pain on urination, pain over one or both kidneys, and fever. But most of the time these infections cause no symptoms at all. More than 30 percent of women 70 years of age or older have symptomless urinary tract infections, as do 10 percent of men in this age group. Because they don't need to be treated, there is no reason to do urine cultures for adults who have no symptoms. Pregnant women, however, are at risk for symptomless urinary tract infections that can turn into symptomatic disease—a complication for the mother, and a potentially serious threat to the fetus.

The two most common sites of urinary tract infection are the bladder (cystitis) and the kidneys (pyelonephritis). Bladder infections are relatively easy to cure, usually with three to five days of antibiotic treatment. Kidney infection is both more serious and more difficult to eradicate, generally requiring two weeks of an antibiotic. The choice of which antibiotic to use became problematic in recent years because of a highly antibiotic-resistant strain of *Escherichia coli*, which has now spread around the world. In this case, as in so many others, antibiotic resistance is fueled by the overuse and misuse of antibiotics—for example, in nonpregnant adults with symptomless urinary tract infections.

Immunization

> Having children made us look differently at all these things that we take for granted, like taking your child to get a vaccine against measles and polio.
>
> Melinda Gates, Bill and Melinda Gates Foundation

Not everyone shares doctors' enthusiasm for vaccines. In 1975, when I was an infectious diseases fellow, I was involved in the care of a 63-year-old farmer who died of tetanus (lockjaw). Three months earlier, another farmer, of about the same age, came close to dying as a result of this same bacterial infection, so I was shocked when the wives of both patients told me that there would be little or no interest if I were to launch a tetanus vaccination campaign in their community. Neither of these farmers had been vaccinated against tetanus, even though farmers are at increased risk because they are exposed to soil, which is where the tetanus bacterium lives.

Because of routine immunizations, Americans rarely contract (or even hear much about) tetanus. In the United States there are only about 100 cases annually. Globally, however, more than one million cases occur each year, and the annual death toll approaches 500,000. The vast majority of these cases occur in developing countries, among nonimmunized people.

It is impossible to exaggerate the benefit of immunization. In the span of my medical career, an immunization campaign eradicated one infection (smallpox) and an active campaign is close to eradicating another (polio). The last naturally occurring case of smallpox, caused by variola virus, was in Somalia in 1977. In 1980, smallpox was officially declared as having been eliminated from the face of the earth. The fact that smallpox killed 300 to 500 million people in the twentieth century alone underscores the magnitude of this triumph.

The last case of polio in the Western Hemisphere, due to the wild-type poliovirus, was diagnosed in 1994. Following a coordinated campaign by the World Health Organization, the United Nations Children's Fund, and Rotary International, annual cases of polio worldwide have plummeted by 99 percent. In 1988, there were 350,000 cases of polio; in the twenty-first century, only about

1,000 cases of polio occur each year. A virus that caused fearsome epidemics throughout the first half of the twentieth century will soon be eliminated through immunization.

Cases of whooping cough (pertussis) are currently on the rise throughout the United States and other areas of the world, though it is not entirely clear why this is happening. DTaP, the vaccine used to prevent pertussis, contains a combination of bacterial products, including aP (acellular pertussis). This is a relatively new vaccine, and some doctors worry that, although it is safer than the old whooping cough vaccine, it may not be as effective. Because many of the recent cases of pertussis occurred in nonvaccinated children, it may be that parents' fear of vaccine side effects has played a role in the resurgence of this illness.

The issue of mandatory vaccination has always ignited passionate debate—a debate that goes back to the Puritans. The clash between opponents and advocates is often rooted in different views about personal freedom versus protection of the general public.

Before a vaccine was invented for measles, each year there were four million cases of measles in the United States and between 500 and 1,000 deaths from the disease. Unfortunately, false information associating the measles vaccine with autism has led some parents to refuse the measles vaccine for their children. This reaction is typically followed by outbreaks of measles—including hospitalizations and deaths—among unvaccinated children and adults.

While all vaccinations carry some risks, the benefits of preventing the diseases they target far outweigh the risks. Reliable information on the risks and benefits of vaccines can be found on the Centers for Disease Control and Prevention (CDC) website (www.cdc.gov/vaccines/acip.index.html).

Topics Discussed in Rule 6
Fever

> Humanity has but three enemies: fever, famine, and war; of these by far the greatest, by far the most terrible, is fever.
> Sir William Osler, physician, "Father of Modern Medicine"

> Fever is your friend.
> Phillip K. Peterson, physician

Both doctors and patients pay attention when a fever develops. It is both a symptom (feeling hot) and a sign (a high temperature measured on a thermometer). Infants and young children can't articulate when they feel feverish, but when they become fussy, parents automatically feel their forehead or take their temperature to check for fever.

Is fever a foe ("the worst enemy of humanity," according to Sir William Osler) or a friend? Actually, both interpretations are correct. What Sir William Osler referred to as an enemy wasn't fever itself, but its underlying causes. In his era, common causes of fever included typhoid, typhus, smallpox, measles, tuberculosis, and a long list of other infections. The combined number of deaths from these infections far exceeded the casualties of war.

(Historically, infections were the number one cause of death in all wars until World War II, when improved hygiene and vaccines prevented certain infections.)

It wasn't until the 1960s that doctors realized that fever is a mechanism for fighting infections. Some microbes can't stand the heat, and they die at an elevated body temperature. Also, some aspects of the immune system work more efficiently when the body's temperature is increased. This is why fever is a friend.

Though the thermometer was introduced into clinical practice in the nineteenth century, it wasn't until the 1990s that a study was conducted to identify the normal temperature of healthy adults. As a result, we now know that the body's temperature is normally about a degree lower in the morning (when an oral thermometer reading above 99 degrees is considered elevated) than in the late afternoon (when an oral temperature of 100 degrees is considered abnormally high).

Fever is generated by proteins released from the cells of our immune system that have been stimulated by microbes or by other agents. These proteins target an area in the brain that serves as a thermostat. When this thermostat is turned up, a cascade of events occurs that raises body temperature. One such event is chills (shaking muscles generate heat). Another is the sensation of feeling cold, resulting in an intense desire to crawl into bed and get under the covers to raise our temperature.

Although infectious agents are the most common cause of fever, people who have autoimmune diseases (such as lupus and rheumatoid arthritis) or some kinds of cancer also can have a fever. Allergies to a variety of substances (most commonly medications) can cause fevers as well.

With so many diseases that can cause a fever, how does a doctor determine the cause? Your doctor takes your medical history—or, to put it another way, you tell the doctor your story. Other symptoms can also help point to the diagnosis: cough or sore throat (respiratory tract infection), diarrhea or vomiting (gastrointestinal tract infection), headache and confusion (nervous system infection), painful urination (urinary tract infection), and so on. What is called your "exposure history" can also be important. This includes your exposures to other people with similar symptoms (many infections are contagious), suspicious foods (in the case of gastrointestinal tract infections), animals, medications, sexual activity, and travel.

As soon as your doctor has a good idea of what is causing your fever, he or she will decide what, if any, laboratory tests will help establish the diagnosis. Tests might include a blood test to check your white blood cell count, cultures of your blood and/or urine, or an x-ray. The goal is to get the right diagnosis quickly with the fewest tests.

Dengue

> Dengue fever sounds scary because the word "dengue" has a scary sound. For Florida the infection rate is low, and people that do get infected are not getting very sick.
>
> FOX News

Dengue is caused by any one of four closely related viruses. In the past decade, dengue has emerged as a major public health problem throughout Africa, Asia, Latin America, and the Caribbean.

More than fifty countries in these areas have reported dengue in recent years. More than one million cases of dengue occur annually worldwide, with about 20,000 deaths each year attributed to this infection.

Dengue viruses are transmitted by two species of mosquitoes prevalent in the tropics and also found in the southeastern United States. Outbreaks of dengue were first observed in the United States in Brownsville, Texas, in 2005. And in 2009, the first cases of dengue that were transmitted by mosquitoes within the United States were reported in Key West, Florida. Because no antiviral treatment exists, prevention is essential. Use mosquito spray when traveling in these areas.

The most severe form of this disease, dengue hemorrhagic fever, can be fatal. However, most infected individuals suffer from a milder form of disease, called dengue fever (DF). In addition to fever, people who have DF may have symptoms of headache, pain behind the eyes, and/or pain in joints, muscles, or bones. The deep bone pain is so severe that dengue is often referred to as "break-bone fever." The illness usually subsides in about ten days. The good news is that a promising vaccine is on the horizon, one that protects against three of the four dengue virus strains.

Topics Discussed in Rule 7
Endocarditis
Endocarditis is an inflammation of the lining of the inside of the heart, most commonly due to an infection of one or more of the four heart valves. The most common symptoms associated with endocarditis are prolonged fever, loss of appetite, weight loss, fatigue, and joint pain. The discovery of a new heart murmur is the

most meaningful physical sign of endocarditis. The diagnosis is established by the culturing of blood samples and special heart-imaging procedures.

The best example of why antibiotics are considered miracle drugs is their impact on endocarditis. Before penicillin was available, *everyone* who got endocarditis died. Now, with the use of penicillin and other antibiotics, most patients survive.

The reason for the high mortality of endocarditis is the location of the infection. When bacteria or fungi get into a heart valve, cells of the immune system can't reach them. Without antibiotic treatment, the valve eventually falls apart, or another fatal complication ensues, such as a stroke or an irregular heart rhythm.

For endocarditis to develop, a microbe must first get into the bloodstream. Microbes can enter the bloodstream through a break in the skin caused by a wound or by intravenous injection of drugs, if people share needles. Bacteria also sometimes enter the bloodstream during dental surgery. If a heart valve is damaged by rheumatic fever in childhood or by the aging process, or if an artificial valve (prosthesis) is in place, the risk of infection is increased. This is why dentists prescribe an antibiotic for patients with damaged or prosthetic heart valves before dental surgery.

Even with antibiotic treatment, however, bacterial endocarditis remains potentially lethal. This usually is related to the destruction of a heart valve, resulting in rapid, uncontrollable heart failure. Because of this risk, cardiac surgeons are notified as soon as a diagnosis of endocarditis is made. When a heart valve does fall apart, emergency replacement with a prosthetic valve needs to be done, and needs to be done quickly.

Cytomegalovirus Infection

CMV is the most common congenital (present at birth) infection in the U.S.
> **Centers for Disease Control and Prevention**

In the past several decades, cytomegalovirus (CMV) has reigned supreme as the most common culprit for causing infections in people who receive organ and bone marrow transplants. It is also the most common virus that babies are born with in the United States.

Between 50 and 80 percent of healthy adults in the United States are infected with CMV but have no symptoms. We know that CMV can be transmitted through sexual contact, blood transfusions, and transplanted organs, but most of the time it is not clear how the virus is picked up. CMV can lie dormant in the body for years. But if the immune system is impaired by an HIV infection or by drugs given to prevent the rejection of a transplanted organ, CMV can reactivate from a dormant state and cause serious (or even fatal) disease of the lungs, gastrointestinal tract, or nervous system.

The brain of the developing fetus is especially susceptible to damage by CMV, and CMV is a common cause of congenital disease—disease that is present at birth. About 1 in 150 children are born with congenital CMV infections every year in the United States. In fact, congenital brain disease caused by CMV is more common than fetal alcohol syndrome and Down syndrome. Congenital CMV infection is also the most common cause of hearing loss in children in the United States.

About 1 to 4 percent of uninfected women acquire CMV infection during pregnancy. It is this so-called primary infection that puts a fetus at risk of congenital CMV infection.

Given all this, it is no surprise that many researchers are working on development of an effective vaccine for CMV.

Infections in Day Care Centers

> Generally infants and toddlers in day care have a new viral infection about every three to four weeks.
>
> **Dennis Clements, physician**

Up to seven million day care-related infections occur in the United States each year. Respiratory infections, diarrheal diseases, hepatitis, and CMV infection pass from child to child (and from child to adult) in day care settings. This is a serious public health issue. The CDC website provides authoritative information on preventing and dealing with infections in day care centers (www.cdc.gov/flu/protect/stopgerms.htm).

The keys to preventing infection are good hygiene (especially hand washing) and making sure your child's immunizations are up to date.

Topics Discussed in Rule 8
Influenza

> Influenza pandemics must be taken seriously, precisely because of their capacity to spread rapidly to every country in the world.
>
>   Margaret Chan, Director-General, World Health Organization

> We have to acknowledge the limits of these vaccines, because that continues to be the major barrier to investment in new vaccines.
>
>   Michael T. Osterholm, Director, Center for Infectious Diseases Research and Policy, University of Minnesota

Every year, about 36,000 Americans die of influenza, and 114,000 are hospitalized because of this infection. A large majority of the people who die of influenza are over 65 years of age. A recent carefully done meta-analysis of randomized clinical trials of the efficacy of influenza vaccine suggests that it protects only 59 percent of individuals between 18 and 65 years of age. The evidence that it works in older adults is less clear. But one thing this study made perfectly clear is that we need a better vaccine for this extremely important infection.

October 2009 was the beginning of the second wave of H1N1 influenza virus. Fortunately, by August of 2010, the H1N1 influenza pandemic was over. Initially, it looked as if H1N1 influenza virus could cause a catastrophic loss of life similar to that of the 1918 influenza pandemic, which killed more than 50 million people worldwide. Fortunately, that did not happen: the global deaths from the H1N1 pandemic are estimated at between 284,500 and 579,000.

Influenza viruses circulate widely among birds and pigs. When a new strain appears in humans, it usually contains bits of one of these animal viruses. H1N1 influenza virus was unique in that it contained bits and pieces of bird, swine, and human flu viruses.

In 2011, another influenza strain, called variant H3N2, began circulating in pigs. This virus is genetically related to H1NI influenza virus. By mid-2012, more than 150 cases of variant H3N2 influenza had been reported in humans, most of them in children who had contact with pigs, often at county fairs. Fortunately, their illnesses were generally mild, and no instances of human-to-human transmission have been identified—so far.

Another unusual feature of H1N1 influenza was that, in contrast to almost all seasonal flu epidemics, children and young adults were the hardest hit. Ordinarily, adults over 64 are most likely to die of influenza. (These older adults account for 80% to 90% of all deaths from seasonal flu.) It appears that older adults had some protective immunity against H1N1 from an earlier influenza virus that circulated before 1957.

One of most disconcerting questions raised by the H1N1 influenza pandemic is this: how and why did this novel strain of influenza emerge so unexpectedly? At the time H1N1 appeared, public health experts were worried mainly about another influenza virus—H5N1 or "bird flu."

> Prediction is very difficult, especially about the future.
>
> Niels Bohr, physicist

At about the time I began my infectious diseases training, in 1975, the surgeon general of the United States, William Stewart, declared the war on infections over. He could not have been more wrong.

Less than twenty years later, the Institute of Medicine (IOM) published a report titled *Emerging Infections: Microbial Threats to Health in the United States*. This 1992 report alerted the U.S. Congress to a serious crisis caused by emerging and reemerging infections in the United States. In 2003, a second IOM report, *Microbial Threats to Health: Emergence, Detection, and Response*, highlighted the global nature of this crisis.

Emerging infections are defined as infections caused by microbes that are new or newly recognized or that reemerged as threats since 1967. At last count, about 175 microbes fit this definition. The H1N1 and H5N1 influenza viruses are among the most recent. Other emerging infections include HIV/AIDS, Legionnaires' disease, Lyme disease, Ebola virus infection, West Nile virus infection, severe acute respiratory syndrome (SARS), and methicillin-resistant *Staphylococcus aureus* (MRSA) infection.

There will surely be others to come, and chances are that no one will accurately predict what the next one will be.

Topics Discussed in Rule 9
HIV Infections

> **No war on the face of the Earth is more destructive than the AIDS pandemic.**
>
> Colin Powell, U.S. Secretary of State

HIV/AIDS is currently the world's leading infectious killer—as of 2010, it had claimed more than 27 million lives. An estimated 2 million people die of HIV/AIDS every year. Being infected with the human immunodeficiency virus (HIV) and developing acquired immunodeficiency syndrome (AIDS) can seriously affect a person's health and can lead to death.

The AIDS epidemic was first recognized in 1981. At the time, a small number of young gay men in California were diagnosed with a rare lung infection (pneumocystosis) or a rare blood vessel malignancy (Kaposi's sarcoma). In 1983, HIV was identified by two French scientists, Luc Montagnier and François Barré-Sinoussi, as the cause of AIDS. No one at the time predicted the devastating effect that the AIDS epidemic would have. Nor could they have predicted that the AIDS epidemic would spread around the world. And no one could have predicted in 1981 that heterosexual women would become the most at-risk group—or that thirty years later we would still lack a vaccine to prevent this disease.

By 2008, 33 million people were living with HIV infections. Over two-thirds of them live in southern and central Africa, where 14 million children have been orphaned because of AIDS.

Everything about HIV is astonishingly bad. One reason a vaccine hasn't been forthcoming is that HIV has the unique capacity to grow within key cells of the immune system (CD4 lymphocytes and macrophages). It is an incredibly simple virus with only nine genes (compared with about 23,000 genes in the human genome). Yet these genes can mutate rapidly. This feature of HIV has made development of antiviral drugs particularly challenging. The first widely used anti-HIV drug was zidovudine (AZT). It was approved for use in 1987, but resistance of the virus to AZT quickly became a problem.

To thwart development of viral mutations, cocktails of three or more drugs were made available in 1996. Amazingly, by 2012, twenty-six of these new drug combinations were approved for treatment of HIV infection. These antiviral combinations, called highly active antiretroviral therapy or HAART, have revolutionized the treatment of HIV infection—in countries that can afford these expensive agents. Following the advent of HAART, the annual death rate due to AIDS in the United States plummeted: in 1994, 48,371 deaths were attributed to AIDS; by 1997, AIDS-related deaths fell to 21,399, a decline of more than 50 percent.

The CD4 lymphocyte count of HIV-infected patients is monitored as the main guide to when to start treatment. One approach is to treat early—even when the CD4 lymphocyte count is relatively high. But this places individuals at risk of years of potential side effects from the drugs in the HAART regimen. Waiting until the CD4 count is low, however, delays the benefits of HAART in stopping the destructive influence of the virus on the immune system. Most patients do not start therapy until the CD4 cell count drops below 500. Recent studies, however, suggest that therapy is beneficial at any CD4 count.

Since the introduction of HAART in 1996, not only has the mortality of HIV/AIDS plummeted but the causes of death have changed. Prior to HAART, the main cause of death was opportunistic infections—infections caused by microbes that take advantage of impaired immunity. Because HAART reduces, though does not totally eliminate, HIV, the immune system recovers considerably. Consequently, in the HAART era, people who have HIV infection now die mainly of heart disease and cancer, just like people who aren't infected with HIV.

Despite incredible advances in the treatment of HIV infection, much work remains to be done. About 44 percent of people needing treatment still do not get it. AIDS remains the world's leading cause of death for women of reproductive age; most of these deaths are in Africa. Even in the United States, more than 800,000 people aren't benefiting from life-saving drugs. The CDC attributes this to the estimated 20 percent who are infected with HIV but don't know it. Also, only two-thirds of people who are diagnosed with HIV see a doctor. Poverty and lack of insurance appear to be the main barriers.

HPV Infections

Harald zur Hausen, a German virologist, is credited with the discovery that human papillomavirus (HPV) causes cervical cancer. Subsequently, HPV was found also to be a cause of anal cancer. The incidence of anal cancer has increased significantly in recent years. Men who have sex with men are at increased risk, and if

> Genital human papillomavirus (also called HPV) is the most common sexually transmitted infection (STI).
>
> **Centers for Disease Control and Prevention**

these men have HIV infection they are at even greater risk of developing anal cancer.

Men who are infected with HIV are screened for early evidence of HPV-induced changes in anal epithelial cells, which can be early signs of cancer. Early treatment of such lesions can prevent metastatic disease from developing.

The good news is that there is now an effective HPV vaccine that is recommended for all 11- and 12-year-old girls and boys. Vaccination of males will help prevent sexual transmission of HPV to females, thereby reducing their risk of cervical cancer.

Topics Discussed in Rule 10
Chronic Fatigue Syndrome

> Fatigue is the best pillow.
>
> **Benjamin Franklin, Founding Father**

My colleagues and I established the University of Minnesota's chronic fatigue syndrome research program in 1988—the same year the formal definition of CFS appeared in the medical literature.

CFS is a disorder of unknown cause that is characterized by disabling fatigue for at least six months. Typically, the fatigue is made worse by physical activity and is not relieved by sleep. Other symptoms include muscle or joint pains, headaches, difficulty concentrating, and memory problems.

To diagnose CFS accurately, a long list of medical conditions associated with fatigue must first be excluded, such as disorders of the thyroid or adrenal glands, cancer, lupus, rheumatoid arthritis, multiple sclerosis, and chronic heart, liver, kidney, or lung disease. (For people who have some of these disorders, such as cancer and multiple sclerosis, fatigue is their main symptom.) These diseases are ruled out by checking for abnormalities in physical exams or lab tests—that is, looking for *signs* of disease. Part of the frustration of people who have CFS is that there are no diagnostic signs for the disease—only symptoms.

CFS usually begins with an illness that acts like an acute viral infection. In 1988, we hypothesized that CFS is triggered by an infectious agent that results in an activated immune system. We thought that certain kinds of proteins (called cytokines) released from activated immune cells were responsible for the symptoms. This hypothesis was shared by other research groups in the United States and around the world. But now, twenty-five years later, we're still not sure about this.

By 1988, Epstein-Barr virus (EBV), the cause of infectious mononucleosis, had been ruled out as *the* cause of CFS. In the past several years, two other viruses, murine leukemia virus-related virus (XMRV) and a similar murine leukemia virus, were implicated by two research groups. However, their findings haven't been replicated by other investigators.

Since 1988, more than 3,500 papers have been published on

CFS or chronic fatigue, yet we still don't know what causes it. Despite this impressive research effort, CFS remains an idiopathic disorder—meaning that the cause is unknown.

Three things became clear to us as soon as we established our research program in 1988. First, CFS is a real illness, and it can be severely disabling. Second, although about 20 percent of our patients recovered, most CFS patients need help dealing with a chronic illness. Third, like all patients, those who suffer from CFS need a doctor who listens, asks about their concerns, and advocates on their behalf.

About the Author

Phillip K. Peterson, M.D., is a professor of medicine and an infectious disease specialist at the University of Minnesota Medical School. He is a fellow of the American College of Physicians and of the Infectious Diseases Society of America. Because many infections are public health threats, and many are linked to animals, he is also on the faculties of the University of Minnesota School of Public Health and the College of Veterinary Medicine. Dr. Peterson also has served as an internist and infectious disease consultant at the University of Minnesota Medical Center and Hennepin County Medical Center, both in Minneapolis, Minnesota.